Cost Analysis, Cost Recovery, Marketing, and Fee-Based Services

*A Guide for the
Health Sciences Librarian*

About the Editor

M. Sandra Wood is Head, Reference, The George T. Harrell Library, The Milton S. Hershey Medical Center, The Pennsylvania State University, Hershey, PA 17033. She holds the academic rank of Associate Librarian. Ms. Wood received an M.L.S. from Indiana University and an M.B.A. from the University of Maryland. She is a member of Beta Phi Mu, International Library Science Honor Society, and Beta Gamma Sigma, National Honorary Society for Business Studies. She is the editor of *Medical Reference Services Quarterly,* actively participates in the Medical Library Association and Special Libraries Association, and is the author of numerous journal articles.

Cost Analysis, Cost Recovery, Marketing, and Fee-Based Services

A Guide for the Health Sciences Librarian

M. Sandra Wood, Editor

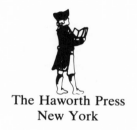

The Haworth Press
New York

Cost Analysis, Cost Recovery, Marketing, and Fee-Based Services: A Guide for the Health Sciences Librarian is a monographic supplement to the journal *Medical Reference Services Quarterly*, Volume 4, 1985. It is not supplied as part of the subscription to the journal, but is available from the publisher at an additional charge.

The Haworth Press, Inc., 28 East 22 Street, New York, NY 10010

Library of Congress Cataloging in Publication Data
Main entry under title:

Cost analysis, cost recovery, marketing, and fee-based services.

   Includes bibliographies and index.
   1. Medical libraries—Costs. 2. Medical libraries—Fees. 3. Medicine—Information services—Costs. 4. Medicine—Information services—Fees. I. Wood, M. Sandra.
Z675.M4C69 1985   026'.61'0681   85-888
ISBN 0-86656-353-9

CONTENTS

V. ANNOTATED BIBLIOGRAPHY

Acknowledgements

I am grateful to the many authors who contributed their time and effort to this supplement and without whom the project could not have been completed. I would also like to acknowledge the contributions of the staff of The George T. Harrell Library, in particular Virginia A. Lingle and Joan L. Bernardo, for their editorial and production assistance.

M. S. W.

Introduction

According to Naisbitt in his book, *Megatrends,* one of the ten trends that are transforming our lives is the shift from an industrial society to an information society. Information is a multi-billion dollar business. It is a real, marketable commodity, as evidenced by the willingness of consumers to pay for fast, accurate and relevant information. The rapid growth of the information business, with the resultant information services and information brokers, and the development of new technologies affecting delivery of these services, raise questions as to how libraries will operate in this new marketplace.

Funding for libraries during the 1970s and early 1980s has not kept pace with the increased amount of information available. Access to the new technologies, such as computerized information retrieval, full-text online, improved telefacsimile transmission, electronic publishing, and electronic mail, all implies additional expenses for libraries over and above traditional costs for books and journals. Libraries wishing to provide access to these services, some of which might be considered individualized or customized, have frequently chosen to charge patrons for these special services since the library budget cannot absorb the costs. Online searching is an example of one such service, where from the beginning libraries have charged patrons for access to computer generated bibliographies. Often the choice of adding a new service or keeping existing services is dependent on cost recovery. The information society, while providing technologically improved and expanded access to information, creates a dilemma for libraries which must decide on what services to offer and to whom; in other words, the library must decide how to compete in the new information marketplace.

In addition to the new information society, health sciences libraries are influenced by factors and events which are unique to their field. The National Library of Medicine (NLM), a leader in online search services, instituted a charge for its MEDLARS system in 1973. While the system was priced less expensively than most other online databases, the charges represented an initial step on the part of NLM toward cost recovery for its services. During the late 1970s, NLM phased in full cost recovery for document delivery provided through its Regional Medical Library Network, a service which had once been free to regional participants. More recently, a court challenge to its method for recovering costs of the MEDLARS system has generated a closer look at NLM's pricing practices.

Marketplace activities affecting the health care industry as a whole represent another special concern to health sciences libraries. Rapid increases in the cost of health care have resulted in the introduction of the prospective payment system and usage of Diagnosis Related Groups (DRGs), a system which encourages better cost control on the part of hospitals. For hospital libraries, the ability to relate costs of services to patient care becomes important if the library is to maintain its share of hospital funding. Because of these events, health sciences libraries are perhaps more aware of the need for cost recovery than are other types of libraries.

These factors all point to the need for librarians to adopt a more "business-like" approach to the operation of the library. The business aspects of providing information include cost analysis, cost recovery and marketing, all of which are important in the operation of a fiscally sound organization. Libraries, as traditional information providers, are being placed in competition with information brokers and other alternative sources of information; to survive, the library must provide needed services at costs which cover the expenses of providing access to information. A common strategy by libraries is to offer fee-based information services.

Adoption of standard cost accounting procedures by libraries, including establishment of cost centers, would facilitate cost analysis for specific services. Information is not free, and both the users of information and the administrators responsible for the library's budget, must know how much it costs to provide specific services. Cost analysis will improve the allocation of library resources, providing the necessary data to decide which programs or services should be funded. Cost recovery takes cost analysis one step further and looks at methods for generating revenue or funding to recover full or partial costs. For example, once costs are known, a pricing strategy can be developed to recover the costs. Fee-based services provide one alternative for libraries to recover fixed costs or overhead. Pricing is one of the four P's of marketing, the others being product, place and promotion. Once the library decides that it will offer a service, whether free or for a fee, marketing is essential for success of the program.

This supplement gives practical advice on cost analysis, cost recovery and marketing of reference services, and presents both information on how to establish a fee-based information service and examples of successful information service programs. While it is oriented toward health sciences libraries, the concepts presented would be relevant to other special, academic and public libraries.

M. Sandra Wood

Cost Analysis, Cost Recovery, Marketing, and Fee-Based Services

A Guide for the Health Sciences Librarian

I. COST ANALYSIS OF REFERENCE SERVICES

Cost analysis is useful for the evaluation and quantification of reference services. The ability to assign costs to specific services through the use of cost centers facilitates both managerial decision making and pricing strategy. Ultimately, it results in improved allocation of library resources. The overview of cost analysis by Wood emphasizes the management uses of cost analysis and provides basic techniques for performing cost analysis, using online search services as the example. Alligood and Russo-Martin detail their experience with methodology for cost analysis and establishing a pricing structure. Circuit librarian programs are normally operated on a cost recovery basis. Levine explains that a detailed cost analysis is a necessary prerequisite for a circuit program. Partin and Wood describe the use of cost analysis as a managerial decision-making tool to reassess a library's document delivery service.

Cost Analysis of Reference Services: An Overview

M. Sandra Wood

ABSTRACT. Both profit-making and not-for-profit organizations are concerned with cost accounting for management purposes and pricing decisions. Libraries have been slow to adopt cost accounting and cost analysis procedures for routine use in evaluating reference services. This article reviews the literature of cost accounting for reference services, focusing on health sciences libraries; provides definitions of cost accounting terminology; illustrates the use of cost analysis for online search services; identifies uses for cost analysis in libraries; and discusses cost-benefit analysis. The article is intended as an overview for reference librarians.

Businesses usually operate within "generally accepted accounting principles," which consist of practices which have evolved and become standardized over many years. Both profit-making and not-for-profit corporations and organizations are concerned with cost accounting for a variety of administrative purposes ranging from cost control to budgeting to long range planning. Despite the importance of cost accounting and analysis to crucial managerial functions, libraries have been slow not only to adopt cost analysis, but consistent application of cost accounting principles among libraries simply is not practiced. There are several reasons for these inconsistencies. First is that the library, frequently a service department of a larger organization, such as an academic health sciences center, hospital or university, may not have been

M. Sandra Wood is Head, Reference, The George T. Harrell Library, The Milton S. Hershey Medical Center, The Pennsylvania State University, Hershey, PA 17033. She received an M.L.S. from Indiana University and an M.B.A. from the University of Maryland.

The author would like to acknowledge the editorial comments of Kelly Murphy Grotzinger, Janne Hunter, Ellen C. Brassil, Suzanne Shultz, and Virginia Lingle.

3

called upon in past years to detail all of its costs or justify specific programs based on cost-benefit analysis or other similar techniques. Second, the method for deriving the library's budget in one institution will not be the same as in another institution. As a result, cross-institutional comparisons are difficult if not impossible. Library budgets in academic settings have traditionally been based either on subjective judgement or oversimplified formulas.[1] Cost analysis in libraries has been oriented more toward budgeting along organizational lines for the library as a whole rather than gathering cost information for specific services.[2]

Two major forces during the 1970s resulted in a more conscious application of cost accounting to library services. The financial cutbacks in library budgets during the past decade forced the need for financial reassessment and retrenchment. Library budgeting became more important as costs of library materials rose faster than funding; concepts such as zero-based budgeting and cost recovery, traditionally viewed as more appropriate for profit-making corporations, took on new meaning for libraries. Additionally, the controversy over fees for service was fueled with the introduction of online search services, which were introduced from the beginning in many libraries as fee-based services. While vendor costs are similar for all libraries, the choice of what costs to pass on to the patron still is highly dependent on individual library policies and philosophies.

With the exception of online searching, cost analysis of reference services generally has been avoided by libraries. The difficulty of accurately measuring and quantifying reference services is well known,[3,4] and the reluctance of many libraries to approach such cost analysis is understandable. Reference librarians have not thought in terms of the utility of cost accounting. Many don't know how much their services really cost and are frequently intimidated by cost accounting procedures.[5] Cost analysis for a service is more complicated than for a product, and this problem is compounded for reference services where it is exceptionally difficult to quantify data.

This article is intended to provide reference librarians with an overview of cost analysis. It begins with a literature review, emphasizing both health sciences libraries and reference services. Formal definitions of cost accounting terminology will be provided, and uses for cost accounting within libraries will be summarized. Online search services will be used as an example for performing cost analysis, and price setting strategy will be discussed in relation to cost analysis. Only basic techniques will be presented; sources will be suggested for information on more advanced techniques. The article will emphasize cost analysis for decision-making purposes.

REVIEW OF THE LITERATURE

Information about cost analysis in libraries, while still not extensive, has become more prevalent over the past decade. As late as 1983, however, Boyce states that "the literature of cost accounting in libraries can only be characterized as sparse."[6] The literature remains inconsistent in its approach to cost accounting principles and is scattered throughout a variety of sources. With the exception of cost analysis of online services, literature on cost accounting of reference services is almost non-existent; Lopez briefly introduced the topic in 1973 as part of an article on reference measurement.[5]

Academic Studies

A good overview of cost accounting and analysis in university libraries was done at the University of California, Berkeley.[2] At that time (1971), the authors remarked on the inconsistencies among libraries with regard to internal cost accounting. Two other notable cost accounting studies on universities were published by Mount and Fasana in 1972[7] and by Drake in 1977.[8] More recently, Mitchell et al. have published a book that describes a model for cost accounting and details the overall system approach used at the California State University, Northridge.[9] These studies attempted to allocate costs of overall library use to various user segments, but did not approach cost analysis of individual services. The above studies illustrate a primary problem which has been associated with the approach that academic libraries have taken to cost accounting. The difficulty is that the costs associated with library services are viewed as joint or indirect costs for all other departments in the institution,[8] whereas the services themselves should be the object of the cost analysis.

Online Search Services

Online searching has become a major focus for cost analysis because the costs of this service can easily be separated from other library functions. The majority of this literature focuses on the comparison of manual and online literature searching,[10-16] or analyzes online search costs for a specific situation.[17] Unfortunately, many of these studies are based on individualized situations which would not be applicable to other libraries. The literature on cost-effectiveness in online searching was reviewed by Koch in 1982.[18] A variety of sources have identified what costs to include in a cost analysis of online searching,[19-22] but in a more technical and philosophical approach, Boyce suggests a model of cost elements to include for online searching that would allow comparisons between libraries.[6]

From a practical standpoint the most useful article on cost analysis is Drinan's "Financial Management of Online Services—A How-to-Guide."[23] The article discusses the methodology for budgeting and pricing online services, presents formulas for cost analysis, and describes how to calculate fees based on the costs that libraries decide they wish to recover. A detailed cost inventory provides a practical guide for the reference librarian faced with deciding what costs to include in a pricing structure.

Several unique, specialized studies have appeared on cost analysis for online searching. For example, Wish et al. used fixed and variable costs to select the optimal computer terminal,[24] Boyce analyzed the cost-effectiveness of on and offline printing,[25] and Cooper and DeWath analyzed costs when searches were free versus when a fee was charged.[26] These studies can be used as models for libraries wishing to design individual cost analyses.

Health Sciences Libraries

Special libraries, including corporate, specialized academic, and health sciences libraries, have developed solid literature relating to cost accounting. Cost analysis studies have appeared regularly since 1970 in the *Bulletin of the Medical Library Association*. The recent emphasis by the National Library of Medicine on cost recovery both within the Regional Medical Library Network and for the MEDLARS system, and the introduction by the government of diagnosis related groups, have made librarians in health sciences institutions much more aware of the need to recover costs.

One of the greatest difficulties in gathering information for cost analysis is determining labor costs. Generally, salaries and fringe benefits are known and can easily be converted into hourly rates. The difficulty lies in determining the appropriate amount of time that is used to perform work for a particular activity. An early article by Spencer on random time sampling detailed a procedure for gathering and determining unit costs for interlibrary loans.[27] Random alarm mechanisms, used for work sampling in industry, had not previously been employed in a library situation. In 1980 Spencer used random alarm devices as a method of self-observation to determine the time and cost of answering reference questions at the National Library of Medicine.[28] While Spencer's previous study covered overall costs of document delivery, the analysis of reference questions was strictly a time and motion study, making no attempt to include costs for materials. Electronic alarm devices had been used to analyze work activities by Divilbiss and Self, although a cost analysis had not been performed.[29]

In 1971, Lutz published an article on cost analysis of information services in health sciences libraries.[30] The article gives detailed information for cost analysis and provides formulas for determining cost recovery. Cable applied cost analysis to a reference service provided to outside users of the University of Oregon Health Sciences Center Libraries.[31] This analysis was confined to direct costs and did not attempt to include "hidden," or indirect costs. Shirley surveyed academic health sciences libraries to determine costs involved in providing online search services.[20] Costs were divided into production costs, support costs and overhead.

Two studies detail cost allocation for the overall library budget. Lyders et al., have described the method of cost allocation that the Houston Academy of Medicine–Texas Medical Center (HAM–TMC) Library uses to handle the library's fixed support costs.[32] The HAM–TMC Library, part of a multi-institutional health complex, allocates its budget to its member institutions on three factors: a basic factor, a head count factor, and a factor based on library use. Countway Library at Harvard University has also designed a method for recovering costs for library services by developing seventeen cost centers within the library for nineteen services; each affiliated institution is then assessed a fee based on library use.[33]

In a significant article published in 1983, Schultz argues for the establishment of cost centers within medical center libraries, an essential step in performing cost accounting in any organization.[34] Rather than the library being viewed by the organization as a single cost center, divisions within the library, such as reference or circulation, must be viewed as cost centers so that expenses can be charged back to the center which incurs the expense. The establishment of cost centers paves the way for cost recovery for library use.

Most recently, a research study, supported by the National Library of Medicine and the National Science Foundation, was conducted among ninety-five health sciences libraries. The study "provides estimates of the national costs of library services through the three principal services of circulation, reference, and in-house use," but perhaps more importantly, it "establishes a method for obtaining results that can be compared and combined across libraries."[35] The study is analyzed by type of user, service and function for nine classes, or sizes, of libraries.

Building on the basic cost studies in academic libraries, and the cost analysis for online searching, health sciences librarians are beginning to use cost analysis as a mechanism for cost recovery and managerial decision making. Schultz's plea for the use of cost centers and Kantor's cost study, designed to provide comparative cost data for health sciences libraries, are significant in their recognition of the need for standardized cost accounting procedures.

COST ANALYSIS

Cost accounting can be as detailed as one might wish to make it. The subject is a separate discipline within the management field, and the literature fills volumes. The methods described here will be simplified, so as to provide a common, starting ground. The intended application is for librarians to consider cost analysis for evaluation and control of reference services, including online search services, information questions, and document delivery.

Definitions

The terminology of cost accounting is so specific that definitions will be presented first. *Cost* "is a measure of the amount of resources used for some purpose."[36] Measurement implies quantification; therefore, "resources" usually refers only to tangible goods or services which can be monetarily quantified. Costs are generally accumulated for a purpose, which is termed a *cost objective.*

Full cost "is the total amount of resources used for a cost objective."[36] Another useful term to librarians is *cost center* which might be equated to a department or a service. A *cost center* "is a cost objective for which costs of one or more related functions or activities are accumulated."[37] Further, a cost center may be considered an intermediate cost objective, which distinguishes it from the final objective—a product or service. For example, in online searching, the online search service might be considered a cost center, while the search itself would be the cost objective.

Costs are traditionally divided into direct and indirect costs, with direct costs being further divided into material and labor. *Direct costs* "are costs that can be traced to a single cost objective."[36] These costs would include salaries, fringe benefits, materials and resources that can be attributed directly to a program. If the program did not exist, these costs would not be incurred. *Indirect costs* "are elements of cost that are associated with or caused by two or more cost objectives jointly, but that are not directly traceable to each of them individually."[37] The general principle is that indirect costs are allocated to each cost objective based on some equitable method. The *full cost* of a cost objective "is the sum of its direct costs plus an equitable share of indirect costs."[36]

Costs may also be divided into fixed and variable costs. While these terms originate in the economic literature and refer to industrial production levels, they are equally applicable to service industries, including libraries. *Variable costs* "are those that change proportionally with changes in volume, that is, the level of activity."[36] *Fixed costs,* on the other hand, do not vary with the volume or level of production. It must be remembered that fixed costs are only "fixed" for a specified length of time, e.g., a year; in the long run, all costs are variable. "The sum of variable and fixed cost is the total cost."[38] It is important to remember that while direct and indirect costs, and fixed and variable costs, both add up to total costs, they are not the same. Direct costs can be both fixed and variable.

A frequently mentioned term in cost analysis is overhead. "*Overhead cost* includes all indirect production costs, that is, all production costs other than direct material and direct labor."[37] These costs range from supervisors' salaries and salaries of personnel shared by several services, to heating, electricity and maintenance. For the purposes of this discussion, overhead will be equated with indirect costs.

Procedure

As mentioned previously, the process of cost analysis can be as simple or as complicated as the individual wishes or as the situation warrants. General principles will be described here, based on the definitions presented above. More detailed descriptions of the methodologies for cost analysis, including complex formulations, are available elsewhere.[13,14,30]

The first step in cost analysis is to decide what is going to be analyzed, i.e., what is the cost objective? Are you performing a cost analysis on the individual product (a "per item" unit), or is the cost analysis to be performed on the cost center as a whole. This decision may or may not alter the overall costs to be included, but certainly will determine what costs are direct or indirect, fixed or variable.

The next step is to determine what items of cost to include in the analysis. Classifying the items into direct or indirect, and fixed or variable, is a convenient way of categorizing the total costs. The primary object of the analysis is to establish an accurate description of the costs involved in providing the product or service. This step is easier for an activity such as online search services, but more difficult for a service such as answering reference questions. Costs for some library services, such as online search services, have already been detailed in the literature, so that a literature search would be an appropriate starting point for generating ideas. However, since many costs are particular to specific libraries, a group, or departmental, approach for identifying cost items is recommended. Suggested group decision-making techniques include brainstorming and the nominal group technique (a round robin listing of ideas).[39] It is important to include *all* costs, not just those that the library might be considering for cost recovery. Administration, both library and institutional, should be made aware of the full cost of a service. The specific classification for the costs will depend on the cost objective.

Once the items of cost have been determined and classified, the exact methodology of gathering the actual cost information must be decided upon. Some costs will be obvious and easy to collect. For example, for online searching, direct costs such as computer connect time, royalties, communications and offline print charges are detailed in vendor invoices and must simply be totaled. Other costs will be more difficult to determine. In the case of direct labor, the employees' salaries will be known, and the percentage to include for fringe benefits will be available from the institution's personnel office. The difficulty lies in determining the exact amount of time that the employee is engaged in activities related to the cost objective. A common, relatively unsophisticated method for gathering this data is to have the employee, perhaps in conjuction with his or her supervisor, estimate the amount of time. Other methods include random alarm mechanisms and observation.

The most difficult items of cost to determine are the indirect expenses. Overhead figures are frequently available from the institution's administrative offices or from the grants and contracts department. Since the library itself is often included as overhead to other departments, libraries should be cautious in accepting a set figure for institutional overhead without a list of specific costs. In detailing indirect costs for certain reference services, other departments such as cataloging or acquisitions should be considered for inclusion. The purpose and the time available for cost analysis will influence the selection of the appropriate methods for data collection.

It follows that the next step is actual collection of the

data—filling in the "blanks" that have already been established by the previous steps. The methods selected for gathering the data will influence the time and complexity of this step. The data collected must then be categorized and analyzed; division of the costs into direct/indirect and fixed/variable costs will facilitate the analysis. Common practice is to further divide direct costs into materials and labor.

Dependent on the purpose of the cost analysis and the data gathered, the information may result in overall costs for a service (i.e., a cost center), or perhaps in an average "per item" cost. It is important that the costs gathered be useful for decision-making purposes. Cost accounting should be a routine part of budgeting and managerial control, but cost analysis of specific services or products must be purposeful. Data collection in and of itself serves no purposes; ultimately, the importance of cost analysis rests with the use to which it is put.

COST ANALYSIS OF ONLINE SEARCH SERVICES

Online search services are used as an example of cost analysis because the costs are more easily identified than those of other reference services. In fact, Boyce states that online searching does not fit the traditional library budget model because the service is "virtually free of the constraints of the collection."[6] Online bibliographic searching provides a product which is based on user demand. A majority of the direct costs are highly visible because these costs are billed by the vendors and are easily quantified.

The cost items for online search services have been identified in several articles.[6,13,18-23] While there is general agreement over the majority of costs to be included in the analysis, the placement of these cost items into direct/indirect and fixed/variable costs is not consistent. These differences can be attributed to individual library practices and the approach to online searching as either a cost center or a cost objective. While it is not possible to detail costing differences of individual libraries, costs for online search services will be presented here based on the service as a whole and on the individual search.

Online Search Services as a Cost Center

Cost accounting for online search services may be approached as a cost center. Table 1 assigns the elements of cost to standard categories. All of the direct costs, both fixed and variable, can be attributed specifically to the cost center. The variable costs change proportionately with the volume of searches performed, while the fixed costs remain the same over a set period of time (e.g., one year).

The first three items of direct variable costs shown in Table 1 are standard for online searching. The search analyst's salary and fringe benefits are variable for a search analyst who devotes part of the time to searching and part to other reference services; if the search analyst does full-time searching, this becomes a fixed cost.

The direct fixed costs are attributed specifically to the cost center; that is, an expense for these items occurs only as a result of the search service. The costs do not change proportionately with the quantity of searches performed. The placement of supplies in the direct fixed costs section might be debated since the quantity of supplies used will vary with the number of searches requested. However, since supplies are usually ordered in bulk quantity, frequently only once or twice per year, they are considered fixed for that length of time.

Indirect costs (overhead costs) are fixed costs. Many libraries assign an overhead cost in the form of a percentage to public service activities. Administrative personnel within the library's institution should be able to provide relevant figures to allow the library to determine indirect costs.

Based on the costs outlined in Table 1, the calculation of total costs for the service, or cost center, are:

Direct Costs + Indirect Costs = Total Costs

The average cost of an individual search would be determined by taking the total costs and dividing it by the total number of searches.

Online Search Services as a Cost Objective

The items of cost included in treating online search services as a cost objective are the same as for the cost center. In the

TABLE 1

ONLINE SEARCH SERVICES AS COST CENTER

Direct Costs

    Variable

        Online Connect Time Charges

        Telecommunications Charges

        Offline Print Charges

        Search Analyst (if full-time, this becomes a fixed cost)

           Salary

           Fringe Benefits

    Fixed

        Terminal/Equipment (includes rental or purchase, maintenance, depreciation)

        Thesauri/Search Aids

        Training/Continuing Education

        Telephone

        Supplies (paper, search forms, postage, etc.)

        Marketing/Promotion

Indirect Costs (Overhead)

        Utilities

        Physical Space

        Rent

        Insurance

        Clerical Support Staff

        Bookkeeping

        Administration

TABLE 2

ONLINE SEARCH AS COST OBJECTIVE

Direct Costs

    Materials

        Online Connect Time

        Telecommunications

        Offline Print Charges

    Labor

        Salary

        Fringe Benefits

Indirect Costs

    Overhead

    Fixed Costs

        Terminal/Equipment

        Thesauri/Search Aids

        Training/Continuing Education

        Telephone

        Supplies

        Marketing/Promotion

example, the focus is the cost of the search itself and not the cost center, or service, as a whole. Table 2 details the items of cost for the online search or cost objective. All direct costs are variable, changing with each search performed. Direct fixed costs for the cost center are now considered indirect fixed costs for the cost objective, since these costs cannot be attributed specifically to any one search. Instead, they are spread out as indirect costs with a proportion attributable to all searches.

Total cost for the search service as a whole can again be

determined by adding direct and indirect costs. Treating on-line searches as a cost objective, however, facilitates deter-mining a "cost per search." Direct costs plus a "fair share" of the indirect costs equals cost per search. A basic formula for a unit cost is:

$$\text{Direct Costs} + \frac{\text{Indirect Costs}}{\text{Number of Items}} = \text{Per Item Cost}$$

Libraries wishing to establish an equitable service fee to be added to the direct costs for each search would divide the total indirect costs by the number of searches performed, based on data from a specific time period.

As can be seen, the same costs were accumulated for each method of analyzing online search services, but the items of cost were assigned differently based on analyzing the costs of the service as a whole (cost center) or the individual search (cost objective). The decision of which approach to take when evaluating the costs of online search services will depend on the purpose of the analysis.

RATIONALE FOR COST ANALYSIS

The question might be asked, "Why perform cost analy-sis?" For libraries which derive their budget from one source, cost analysis might not appear to have significant benefits. Libraries which draw on multiple sources of fund-ing may have either a set formula for charging back ex-penses, or may have performed overall use studies to deter-mine cost allocation. What is at question here, however, is cost analysis of the actual services that are performed by the library—in particular, reference or public services. Specifi-cally, how much does it cost to provide a service or product? The reasons for cost analysis may be divided into two pri-mary objectives: management or administrative purposes, and cost recovery or pricing decisions. Of the two, the man-agement function is by far the most important; cost account-ing should be an integral part of management regardless of whether cost recovery is an issue.

Management Use of Cost Analysis

The primary purpose for using cost accounting is to provide information that is useful for managerial decision making. Within this context, it is inconceivable that more libraries have not used cost analysis as a routine administrative tool. Management decision areas include: budget preparation; program evaluation or justification of services; staffing; comparison with other libraries, departments or services; communication with administration; and long range planning. All of the management functions are, of course, highly interrelated. These uses for cost analysis are expanded below.

Budget Preparation. Cost analysis, not only of the library as a whole, but of specific departments and services in particular, allows for budget preparation based on program budgeting instead of line itemization of disbursements.[5] Knowledge of both overall costs and individual program costs improves an administrator's ability to allocate library resources effectively. The development of cost centers and the use of standardized cost accounting procedures in libraries is a positive step toward both budget preparation and fiscal control.

Programming. Programming decisions are best made when the true cost of operating a program or service can be determined. Cost analysis can facilitate decisions such as whether to discontinue a service due to low use and high cost, or which program to initiate. The assignment of weighted factors (i.e., how important is this service to the patron or the library?) to specific programs, in conjunction with cost analysis, would enhance the quality and objectivity of the decision. The synergy of services is also a consideration in programming; discontinuing one service or changing the price for that service because it is not "pulling its own weight" might affect another service which is profitable. Programming decisions should be based both on cost and marketing data.

Staffing. Staffing decisions, such as the number of professionals in the reference department, or scheduling for the reference desk, are facilitated when the true cost of providing a service is known. Time and motion studies provide the basis for decisions to change staffing patterns, alter services, or add personnel. For example, a library might find it more cost-effective to hire two part-time reference librarians for peak hours at the reference desk rather than to hire one full-time librarian.

Comparative Data. Establishment of cost centers within libraries and use of standardized cost accounting principles would provide comparative data between departments and services for use within a library and with other libraries. Internally, comparisons and evaluation of services—both public and technical—must be made to determine whether these services should be continued, be modified or be replaced. Cost accounting provides the mechanism for comparison and evaluation.

Just as reference departments have difficulty quantifying their services because of the wide variety of their activities (you can't add apples and oranges), past cost analyses of libraries have not allowed comparison between libraries due to the lack of standardization in both data collection and cost accounting procedures. The recent study by Kantor, referred to earlier in this paper, is a step in the proper direction. Academic health sciences and hospital libraries which perform cost analyses in the manner prescribed by this study can compare their costs for certain services to nationwide cost data for libraries of a similar size. Comparative data provide one mechanism to facilitate cost control and accountability.

Communication. Reference department managers must provide relevant information about their department to their library director, who in turn will communicate this information to the insitution's administration. Administrators, whether university or hospital, are used to speaking in dollar terms. Information is not free and this fact must be communicated to higher administration. Quantifying services into costs will place the cost of information in perspective to other activities in the institution. Another approach is to quantify the benefits of a service. For example, relating online search services to grants received by the institution (searches performed for these individuals contributed to X dollars being received by the institution) makes the service visible to administrators.

Long Range Planning. Long range planning focuses on a strategic approach to planning. Both profit-making and non-profit institutions engage in long range planning, and cost analysis is an important part of the decision making which is necessary for the development and implementation of a strategic plan. In long range planning, budgeting, programming, staffing and communication are synthesized into one purposeful plan; cost analysis is integral to both the planning process and control mechanism.

Pricing Decisions

The second use for cost analysis, as previously mentioned, is to establish fair and equitable prices for products or services. In libraries these decisions primarily relate to public services, although a variety of technical services are provided by larger libraries for a fee or on a contractual basis to smaller libraries. The issues surrounding pricing decisions are complex. For those libraries which do decide to charge for specific services, or who derive their overall funding from multiple sources, some basis must be established on which to charge for the service, or to "charge back" for the funding.

Pricing is one of the four P's of marketing, according to Kotler. An organization which is making pricing decisions must proceed through three stages. It must first determine the pricing objective, which could be maximizing profit, cost recovery, or some other objective. Then, it must determine pricing strategy, which involves one of three bases for pricing: cost-based, demand-based, or competition-based. Finally, it should determine if a pricing change is needed and methods for implementing it.[40]

Pricing Objectives. In establishing its price objectives, a library must consider the overall goals of the institution along with the library's specific needs in establishing pricing policies.[38] While a business's goal may be to maximize profits, libraries may establish objectives such as full cost recovery, recovery of direct variable costs, or recovery of a "reasonable" portion of the costs.

Rarely is there just one pricing objective. Libraries, in assessing pricing policies, may find that their objectives are conflicting. For example, the objective of full cost recovery for online search services may prevent student use of the service because the price is too high. Similarly, a library policy of giving priority to computer search requests from primary clientele versus non-primary clientele may conflict with a policy of non-discriminatory pricing. Full cost recovery may conflict with a library's policy on equal access to information, while recovery of direct variable costs alone may not be adequate to justify providing a service. Pricing remains an individualized decision based on a library's service philosophy and economic realities.

Pricing Strategies. The three primary pricing strategies are cost-based, demand-based, and competition-based. Selection of a pricing strategy follows the establishment of pricing objectives. While more detailed information on these pricing strategies is available elsewhere,[30,36,38,40,41] they are briefly discussed here.

1. *Cost-Based-Pricing.* In cost-based pricing, a library would establish a price for a service based primarily on cost. Perhaps the most common form of cost-based pricing for a non-profit institution is full cost pricing, which is determined by adding all direct and indirect costs. A typical way to determine full costs is to perform a breakeven analysis, which establishes the number of units which must be "sold" to cover costs. This is called the breakeven volume.[40] Drinan illustrates the process of budgeting and pricing for online search services based on estimates of volume of searches.[23]

A variety of cost-based pricing strategies are available including: full cost recovery, partial cost recovery, cost-plus pricing, target-rate-of-return pricing, markup pricing, value-added pricing, and minimum value pricing. The latter, minimum value pricing, "is a method which recovers only those variable costs associated with directly performing the service."[30] This form of pricing, equivalent to the "economic short run," is a common pricing strategy for libraries providing online search services.

2. *Demand-Based Pricing.* Pricing that considers demand as opposed to costs in establishing prices is called demand-based pricing. Basically, this strategy charges "what the market will bear." The price for a product or service should reflect the value that the client perceives it is worth.[38] With demand-based pricing, prices are lowered where demand for a service is weak and raised where demand is high. A form of demand-based pricing would be discriminatory pricing for online search requests where discount rates are given to students to

encourage them to utilize the service. Primary clientele might be charged a rate which would recover direct variable costs plus a portion of direct fixed costs. On the other hand, external users, or non-primary clientele, might be charged a higher rate designed to lessen demand and also to recover full costs. To effectively implement demand-based pricing for reference services, marketing research should be performed; this research would assess such questions as: what services should be offered, to whom should they be offered, where or when they should be offered, and why should they be offered (what purpose do they serve).

3. *Competition-Based Pricing.* With this form of pricing, a library would establish prices based on "what other producers of the same product or service are charging."[38] A favorite type of competitive strategy is imitative pricing, where the pricing depends on what major competitors (other libraries) are charging. Three choices exist: charge the same price, charge a higher price, or charge a lower price. Libraries may wish to charge the "going rate" for a service; an example would be to charge the rate established for document delivery in the National Library of Medicine's Regional Medical Library Network.

Price Changing. Libraries which have established prices for services or products should periodically reexamine their pricing objectives and pricing strategies to determine whether a change is warranted. Only three choices are available: a price increase, a price decrease, or the same price. Obviously, any pricing change will increase or decrease demand, dependent on the option selected. Libraries considering implementing a new pricing structure or changing existing prices are encouraged to perform a cost analysis for the service or product. The cost analysis, in conjunction with a reevaluation of library policies and philosophy regarding cost recovery and access to information, will aid in the decision-making process.

COST-BENEFIT ANALYSIS

Generally, costs measure the use of resources. In order for costs to be comparable, they are usually expressed in monetary terms and are gathered for a specific purpose.[37] Too frequently, people think of costs only in terms of price, asking, "How much is this search going to cost me?" Cost accounting and cost analysis translate units of labor or materials into standard costs which can be compared on an equal basis with costs of other services. This is done to provide some means of objectively assessing the service or product.

Despite advocating the use of cost analysis as a means of measuring and evaluating reference services, it must be acknowledged that all costs cannot be quantified or translated into monetary costs. Additionally, cost is not only measurable from the provider's (the library's) viewpoint. The user also bears a private cost of using the library.[42] In addition to price, costs include effort costs, psychic costs, and waiting costs.[40] This may be exemplified by the patron's evaluation of his own time in using a library; it may be both cost-effective and cost-efficient for a user to request a computer search or inhouse photocopying rather than to do his own library work.

Cost-benefit analysis refers to the comparison of the costs of a service or product with the benefits that accrue from the results of having that service performed or product produced. "Cost-effectiveness measures the effectiveness of something relevant to its cost."[4] The costs involved may be both monetary and non-monetary; they refer both to the library's and the library user's costs. Benefits are less easy to quantify than costs and may refer to such vague concepts as "benefits to society" or "public good." In evaluating costs and benefits, it is more relevant to look at "private" costs and benefits, for example, those borne directly by the library or the library user.[42]

Martyn and Lancaster suggest three cost-benefit criteria for information systems: prevention of duplication, saving of research time, and promotion of research efficiency. One way of approaching such an analysis is from the viewpoint of an "opportunity lost." To a library patron who needs certain information immediately for a grant proposal and does not have the time to do his own searching, the price of a computer search does not compare with the grant funding that might be lost if the search were not performed. Similarly, an article which is found through a computer search but which would have been missed via a manual search, may have a value to the patron that exceeds monetary cost. A cost-benefit analysis is thus not complete when approached strictly from the library's perspective; the costs and benefits of the library user should be considered in addition to those of the library. The information itself and the method by which it is obtained each have their own value.[42]

SUMMARY

Cost analysis provides a method for quantifying and evaluating reference services that allows for comparison between services and with other libraries. Adoption of standard cost accounting procedures, including the use of cost centers, is essential to facilitate this comparison. Cost analysis must be purposeful—the two primary purposes being managerial decision making and price setting. The uses for cost analysis range from budgeting and long range planning to staffing and programming. The costs and benefits accruing to both library and user should be considered in any decision resulting from cost analysis. While cost analysis should not be the sole method for evaluation, implementation of cost accounting for reference services as a routine practice provides valuable objective data and is long overdue in many libraries.

REFERENCES

1. Keller, John E. "Program Budgeting and Cost Benefit Analysis in Libraries." *College & Research Libraries* 30 (March 1969) :156–60.

Leimkuhler, Ferdinand F., and Cooper, Michael D. "Cost Accounting and Analysis for University Libraries." *College & Research Libraries* 32 (November 1971):449–63.

3. Lancaster, F. W. *The Measurement and Evaluation of Library Services.* Washington, D.C.: Information Resources Press, 1977.

4. Martyn, John, and Lancaster, F. Wilfrid. "Cost Analysis." In: *Investigative Methods in Library and Information Science: An Introduction,* by John Martyn and F. Wilfrid Lancaster. Arlington, Va.: Information Resources Press, 1981, pp. 175–92.

5. Lopez, Manuel D. "Academic Reference Service: Measurement, Costs and Value." *RQ* 12 (Spring 1973):234–42.

6. Boyce, Bert R. "A Cost Accounting Model for Online Computerized Literature Searching." *Journal of Library Administration* 4 (Summer 1983):43–9.

7. Mount, Ellis, and Fasana, Paul. "An Approach to the Measurement of Use and Cost of a Large Academic Research Library System: A Report of a Study Done at Columbia University Libraries." *College & Research Libraries* 33 (May 1972): 199–211.

8. Drake, Miriam A. "Attribution of Library Costs." *College & Research Libraries* 38 (November 1977):514–9.

9. Mitchell, Betty Jo; Tanis, Norman E.; and Jaffe, Jack. *Cost Analysis of Library Functions; A Total System Approach.* Greenwich, Connecticut: Jai Press, 1978.

10. Bivans, Margaret M. "A Comparison of Manual and Machine Literature Searches." *Special Libraries* 65 (May/June 1974):216–22.

11. Elman, Stanley A. "Cost Comparison of Manual and On-Line Computerized Literature Searching." *Special Libraries* 66 (January 1975):12–8.

12. Calkins, Mary L. "On-Line Services and Operational Costs." *Special Libraries* 68 (January 1977):13–7.

13. Elcheson, Dennis R. "Cost-Effectiveness Comparison of Manual and On-Line Retrospective Bibliographic Searching." *Journal of the American Society for Information Science* 29 (March 1978):56–66.

14. Flynn, T.; Holohan, P.A.; Magson, M.S.; and Munro, J.D. "Cost Effectiveness Comparison of Online and Manual Bibliographic Information Retrieval." *Journal of Information Science* 1 (May 1979):77–84.

15. Cornell, Joseph A. et al. "Cost Comparison of Searching the Iowa Drug Information Service Index Manually and by Computer." *American Journal of Hospital Pharmacy* 38 (May 1981):680–4.

16. Buntrock, Robert E. "Cost Effectivness of On-Line Searching of Chemical Information: An Industrial Viewpoint." *Journal of Chemical Information and Computer Science* 24 (May 1984):54–7.

17. Cooper, Michael D., and DeWath, Nancy A. "The Cost of On-Line Bibliographic Searching." *Journal of Library Automation* 9 (September 1976):195–209.

18. Koch, Jean E. "A Review of the Costs and Cost-Effectiveness of Online Bibliographic Searching." *Reference Services Review* 10 (January-March 1982):59–64.

19. Saffady, William. "The Economics of Online Searching: Costs and Cost Justification." *Library Technology Reports* 15 (September-October 1979):567–653.

20. Shirley, Sherrilynne. "A Survey of Computer Search Costs in the Academic Health Sciences Library." *Bulletin of the Medical Library Association* 66 (October 1978):390–6.

21. Hawkins, Donald T. "Management of an Online Information Retrieval Service." In: *The Library and Information Manager's Guide to Online Services*, edited by Ryan E. Hoover. White Plains, N.Y.: Knowledge Industry Publications, Inc., 1980, pp. 97–125.

22. Atherton, Pauline, and Christian, Roger W. *Librarians and Online Services.* White Plains, N.Y.: Knowledge Industry Publications, Inc., 1977.

23. Drinan, Helen. "Financial Management of Online Services—A How to Guide." *Online* 3 (October 1979) :14–21.

24. Wish, John; Collins, Craig; and Jacobson, Vance. "Terminal Costs for On-Line Searching." *College & Research Libraries* 38 (July 1977):291–7.

25. Boyce, Bert R., and Gillen, Edward J. "Is It More Cost-Effective to Print On- or Offline?" *RQ* 21 (Winter 1981):117–20.

26. Cooper, Michael D., and DeWath, Nancy A. "The Effect of User Fees on the Cost of On-Line Searching in Libraries." *Journal of Library Automation* 10 (December 1977):304–19.

27. Spencer, Carol C. "Random Time Sampling With Self-Observation for Library Cost Studies: Unit Costs of Interlibrary Loans and Photocopies at a Regional Medical Library." *Journal of the American Society for Information Science* 22 (May-June 1971):153–60.

28. Spencer, Carol C. "Random Time Sampling with Self-Observation for Library Cost Studies: Unit Costs of Reference Questions." *Bulletin of the Medical Library Association* 68 (January 1980):53–7.

29. Divilbiss, J.L., and Self, Phyllic C. "Work Analysis by Random Sampling." *Bulletin of the Medical Library Association* 66 (January 1978):19–23.

30. Lutz, Raymond. "Costing Information Services." *Bulletin of the Medical Library Association* 59 (April 1971) :254–61.

31. Cable, Leslie G. "Cost Analysis of Reference Service to Outside Users." *Bulletin of the Medical Library Association* 68 (April 1980):247–8.

32. Lyders, Richard; Eckels, Diane; and Leatherbury, Maurice C. "Cost Allocation and Cost Generation." In: *New Horizons for Academic Libraries,* edited by Robert D. Stueart and Richard D. Johnson. New York: K.G. Saur Publishing, Inc., 1979, pp. 116–22.

33. Rousmaniere, Peter F.; Ciarkowski, Elaine F.; and Guild, Nathaniel. "Bridging the Library Budget Gap; An Approach to Creating Fair User Charges." *College & Research Libraries News* 44 (March 1983):69–71.

34. Schultz, Claire K. "Establishing Cost Centers Within Libraries of Medical Centers." *Bulletin of the Medical Library Association* 71 (January 1983):1–5.

35. Kantor, Paul B. "Cost and Usage of Health Sciences Libraries: Economic Aspects." *Bulletin of the Medical Library Association* 72 (July 1984):274–86.

36. Anthony, Robert N., and Herzlinger, Regina E. *Management Control in Nonprofit Organizations.* Revised Edition. Homewood, Il.: Irwin, 1980.

37. Anthony, Robert N., and Reece, James S. *Accounting; Text and Cases.* 6th edition. Homewood, Il.: Irwin, 1979.

38. Zais, Harriet W. "Economic Modeling: An Aid to the Pricing of Information Services." *Journal of the American Society for Information Sciences* 28 (March 1977):89–95.

39. Huber, George P. *Managerial Decision Making.* Glenview, Il.: Scott, Foresman and Company, 1980.

40. Kotler, Philip. *Marketing for Nonprofit Organizations.* 2nd edition. Englewood Cliffs, N.J.: Prentice-Hall, 1982.

41. Rados, David L. *Marketing for Non-Profit Organizations.* Boston, Ma.: Auburn House, 1981.

42. Braunstein, Yale M. "Costs and Benefits of Library Information: The User Point of View." *Library Trends* 28 (Summer 1979):79–87.

Cost Analysis of Online
Search Services in an
Academic Health Sciences Library

Elaine C. Alligood
Elaine Russo-Martin

ABSTRACT. The Claude Moore Health Sciences Library, a medium-sized academic health sciences library, serves the University of Virginia Medical and Nursing Schools. Fully cognizant of the high costs and the utility of its online search services, the Library initiated a study of the direct and indirect search service costs, the charges to patrons, and the actual cost recovery. Further, the Library's philosophy of charging, the staff's and user's billing requirements and preferences were examined, along with the impact of current trends in online search services. As a result, the Library developed a methodology for analyzing costs and setting a search rate structure consistent with Library and user needs.

INTRODUCTION

Call it fee-for-service, or institutional survival—whatever the perspective, old notions of service for service's sake are being modified or replaced by calls to "pay as you go," to

Elaine C. Alligood is User Education Officer for EMBASE, Excerpta Medica online database, North American Database Department, Elsevier Science Publishing Company, 52 Vanderbilt Avenue, New York, NY 10017. At the time of the study she was Assistant Director for Public Services, The Claude Moore Health Sciences Library, University of Virginia, Charlottesville, VA 22908. She received her M.L.S. from the University of Maryland.

Elaine Russo-Martin is Assistant Head of Reference for the Paul Himmelfarb Health Sciences Library, George Washington University Medical Center, 2300 Eye Street, NW, Washington, DC 20037. At the time of the study she was a reference librarian at The Claude Moore Health Sciences Library. She received her M.S.L.S. from Catholic University.

The authors wish to acknowledge the assistance of Lorraine Frye and Jeffrey Gold in the preparation of this manuscript.

27

recover in some way the actual costs to academic health sciences libraries of online searches. The Claude Moore Health Sciences Library, an example of a library in this situation, is a medium-sized academic health sciences library, serving an approximate user population of 4000 faculty, staff and students within the University of Virginia Schools of Medicine and Nursing. The Library's mission is to provide information resources and services needed to fulfill the medical center's fundamental educational, patient care, research and public service goals. Open sixteen hours a day, the Library is staffed with eleven FTE professionals and nineteen support staff. Professional reference services, including online searching, are available from 8:00 a.m. to 6:00 p.m. Monday through Friday. The Library maintains subscriptions to all major indexes including *Index Medicus, Science Citation Index, Psychological Abstracts, Biological Abstracts, Cumulative Index* to *Nursing and Allied Health Literature, International Nursing Index,* and *Hospital Literature Index.* In addition to printed sources, the Library is equipped with Texas Instruments 820 and 745 terminals, and a Digital Equipment Corporation DECwriter LA120 terminal. Although The Claude Moore Health Sciences Library primarily performs health and basic sciences subject searches, searches in other subject areas such as education and the social sciences are conducted. Search requests by the Medical Center community are accepted, regardless of subject or availability elsewhere. At the time of the study, spring 1982, four reference librarians were performing 333 searches a month, using the four major online vendors: BRS, NLM, SDC, and DIALOG.

Historically, online searches were first performed at The Claude Moore Health Sciences Library free of charge, and somewhat later a minimal flat rate of $2.50 was imposed which remained in effect until September 1982. At the time, the Library, as a matter of policy, required recovery of only a portion of direct search costs by imposing a minimal flat rate and subsidizing the remaining costs. The Library maintained this static flat rate while costs of providing online search services increased. Due to the Library's low charges for searches, cost recovery was so low that by 1981, total direct search costs were 53 percent greater than actual recovery. In 1982, total direct costs were 59 percent greater. Library managers were concerned over this cost recovery gap. If the Library continued subsidizing online search services at this escalating rate, both staff and budget would be so overloaded as to inhibit development and provision of other, equally important reference services.

Since 1974, there had been no formal evaluation of online search services. The lack of current data, and the pressing need to identify and contain costs led the Library staff to undertake a detailed study of online search services to analyze and set fees consistent with the institution's mission of service.

A survey of the literature revealed that studies of online search costs are usually one of three types: (1) comparison of manual search costs with online search costs; (2) theoretical discussion of "fee versus free" issues; and (3) cost analysis of computer search services in order to set a fee. Calkins,[1] Elchesen,[2] and Elman[3] compared the cost effectiveness of manual versus online searching. Although all reported "cost per search" data, none provided significant cost accounting detail. Still, these studies are noteworthy for their methodologies and provide a framework for later "cost per search" research.

Articles from the 1970s primarily focused on "fee-for-service" issues, especially in the public library. In 1974, Blake and Perlmutter[4] warned against user fees, saying "User fees will ultimately create more problems, and more serious problems than they can ever solve in libraries supported by public funds." Later articles studied the impact of imposing fees for online searching on patron demand for the service.[5] By 1977, a survey of 708 United States and Canadian health sciences libraries revealed that over one-half of the respondent institutions charged for online searching.[6]

Little, however, has been written about the methodology for setting a fee for computer search services based upon a cost accounting analysis of a library's costs in providing service. An early Cooper and DeWath[7] study examined the cost of a search by measuring "out of pocket" expenses such as connect time, royalty charges and offline prints. The absence of figures separating out telecommunications charges, however, was a major omission in the study. Atherton and Christian[8] are quick to point out that an online search does not begin and end at the terminal, and urge librarians to consider staff time and overhead charges when determining the budget. Anthony,[9] Shirley,[10] and Boyce[11] provide very detailed lists of categories associated with online searching costs, including such generally ignored items as manuals and searcher training, in order to calculate realistic "cost per search" data. Anthony[9] and Shirley[10] go one step further by discussing factors to consider when deciding which costs to pass on to the user and which costs are to be subsidized by the library, and then determination of fees based on these factors.

METHODOLOGY

The calculations of actual costs at The Claude Moore Health Sciences Library were developed using the work of Shirley[10] and Martyn[12] with further refinement and definition inspired by the articles of Boyce[11] and Anthony.[9] Straightforward, clearly defined cost categories were essential and enabled staff to identify all cost components. For this study, "cost" is defined as the expenditure of various resources in providing a service.[12] Direct or calculable costs are incurred in the course of carrying out the operation of the service. Indirect or overhead costs, incurred on a continuing basis, are not directly associated with a particular operation. Total cost of a service equals the sum of direct and indirect costs.[12] Based on Shirley's 1977 paper, online search service costs divide into four categories,[10] as illustrated in Table 1. Table 2 shows direct costs for production. Categories two, three, and four as illustrated in Table 3 are indirect costs.

1. *Production Costs.* Production costs are those costs directly related to the production of a computer search. For this study, they were defined as connect time, network communications costs, database royalties, offline and online printing charges, and the direct personnel costs for the searcher's time from the presearch interview to the conclusion of the online search process.
2. *Non-personnel Support Costs.* These costs include terminals, maintenance, paper, continuing education classes, database manuals, and all local telephone charges.
3. *Online Support Costs.* The use of online services for purposes other than patron-requested searches, such as

answering ready reference questions, verifying citations, and accessing the "news" files, are included here.

4. *Indirect Costs.* These are composed of fixed items such as building costs, and a portion of the clerical salaries necessary to support the record keeping, processing, and billing for online search services. Initial searcher training costs are considered indirect costs.

Online search service costs to this Library were computed in a three-part study. Retrospective studies of previous year's and current year's costs to date were performed. The majority of the data was gathered by careful examination of accounting records, and annual and monthly report statistics. The third component required a thorough examination of all online search service related costs by recording charges, costs, and operating times on the search request form for a one-month period. As shown in Table 4 data included presearch time spent in interviewing and strategy formulation, the time the searcher spent online, connect time, database royalties, citation or printing charges, communications costs, total search costs, and finally, charges to the patron. Using the data, all costs except fixed building costs and patron charges (cost re-

TABLE 1

SEARCH SERVICES COSTS

1. Production Costs

    Vendor Costs

    Direct Personnel Costs

2. Non-Personnel Support Costs

3. Online Support Costs

4. Indirect Personnel Costs

TABLE 2

DIRECT COSTS -- PRODUCTION COSTS

Connect Time

Communications Costs

Database Royalties

Printing Charges

Personnel Costs

covery) were computed and compared for each database searched during the three study periods, current month, current year, and year to date.

ANALYSIS

The total per month cost of the three categories of indirect expenses (non-personnel support costs, online support costs, and indirect costs) was obtained by adding together the average monthly costs of each of these "hidden" expenses. By dividing this amount by the number of searches performed per month the indirect costs per search were identified. Production cost per search was found by computing the average vendor charges plus the average direct personnel costs per search. Thus, the actual costs of performing each search equals the production costs per search, plus indirect costs per search.

RESULTS

By comparing the actual cost of an average search with the patron charges recovered the month long study's findings revealed that the Library was subsidizing approximately 84 percent of the cost of a MEDLINE search. In other databases,

TABLE 3

INDIRECT COSTS

NON-PERSONNEL SUPPORT COSTS

    Paper

    Continuing Education

    Database Documentation

    Local Telephone Charges

ONLINE SUPPORT COSTS

    Demonstrations

    ILL Verification

    Ready Reference

    News Files

INDIRECT PERSONNEL COSTS

    Clerical Salaries

    Processing and Billing

    User Education

    Initial Searcher Training

TABLE 4

COST STUDY COMPONENTS*

Communications Costs

Connect Time

Total Citations

Online Charges

Page Charges

Royalties

Total Charges

Charge to the Patron

Presearch Time

*For the study month

the Library was found to have subsidized users 54 percent to 88 percent. The projected subsidy for 1981/82 using July 1981 through March 1982 cost figures was 59 percent, with the previous year's subsidy tallying 53 percent.

Clearly, there was need to adjust the subsidy downward and recover more costs. The next step was to determine which costs would be passed on to the requester and which would be absorbed by the Library. At this time, it is necessary to consider both the Library's philosophy and the different possibilities for devising a rate structure.

Library Philosophy

In 1982 "72% of the 985 publicly supported libraries responding to a recent ALA questionnaire charge fees to some or all of those using their online search services."[13] Is this fee-for-service concept, in practice, a denial of open access to information? The feeling at The Claude Moore Health Sciences Library, in most cases, is that charging for online search services is not denial of access if the print subscriptions are retained. In addition, at the librarian's discretion, searches are performed without charge, or at a reduced rate.

In short, the Library's philosophy is to provide basic reference services without charge to all Library users. For example, there is no charge, nor are there plans to charge, for questions answered quickly, by any method, at the reference desk. Online searching is more than a basic reference service. It is specially tailored to meet the requester's individual needs, and it is performed by the librarian, at the initiation of the requester. Therefore, it is an extraordinary reference service, essential to the complete literature review process at the highest level of biomedical and clinical research. Given the nature and costs of online search services, The Claude Moore Health Sciences Library takes a pragmatic stance toward cost recovery and is compelled to charge for extraordinary services.

To the contrary, some librarians believe that the entire direct cost of performing the online search ought not be passed on to the user. Though not a basic reference service, there are components to the search process that are the very "core task" of the reference librarian's profession.[14] This part of the online search process includes professional-client interaction during the online reference interview, and application of the reference librarian's knowledge and professional expertise to the online search task at hand. The cost of this very critical aspect of online search services is not passed on to the user at The Claude Moore Health Sciences Library. The Library willingly subsidizes a service-oriented approach to online information and its retrieval, but it cannot afford to subsidize all production costs. The new pricing structure reflects this philosophy by passing on vendor production costs, but not searchers' time or indirect costs.

Rate Structure

Rather than change to a variable rate that could prove confusing to a clientele accustomed to a flat rate, it was decided to maintain a flat rate structure designed to recover vendor production costs. Flat fees enable the librarian to inform users of the exact cost of a search, eliminate differing charges for users of the same database, reduce searcher stress, and simplify user's bookkeeping.[15] A flat rate of $15.00 for a 1966 to the present MEDLINE search was set, with flat rates for other databases, e.g., $6.00 for ERIC, $7.00 for PsychINFO, and $8.00 for SCISEARCH.

Despite its advantages, a flat fee structure should be specifically defined for users and reference librarians. Situations occur when the user wants more than a "citations only" search. Sometimes the user requests abstracts. Any library, when setting a flat rate structure, must address these issues. Pricing criteria reflecting The Claude Moore Health Sciences Library philosophy of charging for production costs less the direct personnel costs, non-personnel support costs, and indirect personnel costs were identified as follows:

1. Flat rate charges are for citations only. No more than one hundred citations will be printed without additional charges for online connect time.
2. When abstracts are desired, the charge will be the stated flat rate plus the entire online connect charges. The Reference Department reserves the right to limit the number of abstracts printed online as circumstances warrant.
3. Abstracts printed offline will be charged at the stated flat rate plus the total charges for offline printing. Print charges are database dependent and may vary.
4. When some abstracts are printed online and the rest of the abstracts printed offline, the charge will be the stated flat rate plus all online connect charges plus the total charges for offline printing.

IMPLEMENTATION

Determining the rate is one matter, successfully implementing it is, however, another issue altogether. Consideration must be given to: (1) institutional billing systems; (2) impact on library staff; (3) patron reaction; and, (4) evaluation of the billing system. Institutional billing systems are factors to consider insofar as they will affect how, when, and where the patron will pay for and pick up a search. At The Claude Moore Health Sciences Library patrons pick up and pay for searches in cash or by purchase order during regular library hours. The reference secretary attaches an invoice to the search stating the charges. Circulation staff retain the invoices for monthly billing and/or statistics. As with any new procedure, implementation affects staff workload and work patterns, and of course staff morale. At the Claude Moore Health Sciences Library, Circulation and Reference staff participated in developing a new multipurpose invoice, replacing three separate forms. The new form saves billing time, combines three similar procedures, and lessens staff confusion about which form to use. Since patron reaction is directly influenced by prior and prolonged publicity, The Library produced newsletter articles, announcements attached to searches and request forms, and information sheets at the reference desk to inform patrons over a one-month period of the planned change. The successful implementation of the billing system was evinced by the small number of patron/staff complaints and the minimal number of outstanding bill collection requests issued by the University Treasurer.

FUTURE CONCERNS

In addition to in-house concerns, the effects of future trends in online rate structures must be considered. The most obvious trend is that of charging for the "value" of a retrieval, not merely the online connect time used to accomplish it. New fee schedules introduced recently by the National Library of Medicine and other commercial vendors reflect the shifting policies. Their charges are now being computed by a range of sophisticated algorithms combining telecommunications, online time, the amount of material printed (citation charges), keystrokes, and central processing unit time. It remains to be seen how these charges will affect any library's pricing structure given the new, larger number of variables that must be considered by an institution in developing a viable online search rate structure. Indeed, anticipating the impact of complex vendor pricing structures is making life difficult for most library planners. The probable result for The Claude Moore Health Sciences Library, and no doubt, other libraries of a similar kind is a "show cost" recovery system which will charge the patron for the direct search costs displayed by the system at the end of a search. Subsidies will likely take the form of discounts or dollars off for various user categories.

A second trend, user friendly searching within the personal computer market, has kindled the curiosity of many library users for performing their own searches. What is the role, then, for the library and librarian in this virtual information explosion? Should the library provide and support these systems for patrons? If so, ought the library charge? How will such a service affect traditional online search services currently in place? These sorts of questions address fundamental tenets of librarianship outside the scope of this paper. Each library and librarian, however, confronting such issues in the near future, will need to be fully prepared to deal effectively with the powerful potential presented by these new developments in online search services.

REFERENCES

1. Calkins, Mary L. "Online Services and Operational Costs." *Special Libraries* 66 (January 1977):13–7.

2. Elchesen, Dennis R. "Cost-Effectiveness Comparison of Manual and Online Retrospective Bibliographic Searching." *Journal of the America Society for Information Science* 29 (March 1978):56–66.

3. Elman, Stanley A. "Cost Comparison of Manual and On-Line Computerized Literature Searching." *Special Libraries* 66 (January 1975):12–8.

4. Blake, Fay M., and Perlmutter, Edith L. "The Rush to User Fees: Alternative Proposals." *Library Journal* 102 (October 1977):2005–7.

5. Huston, Mary M. "Fee or Free: The Effect of Charging on Information Demand." *Library Journal* 114 (September 1979):1811–4.

6. Werner, Gloria. "Use of On-Line Bibliographic Retrieval Services in Health Sciences Libraries in the United States and Canada." *Bulletin of the Medical Library Association* 67 (January 1979):1–14.

7. Cooper, Michael D., and DeWath, Nancy A. "The Cost of On-line Bibliographic Searching." *Journal of Library Automation* 9 (September 1976):195–209.

8. Atherton, Pauline, and Christian, Roger W. *Librarians and Online Services.* White Plains, NY: Knowledge Industry Publications, Inc., 1977.

9. Anthony, Susan Shelly. "Incremental Charges for Online Services: An Analysis." *National Online Meeting Proceedings, 1981,* Martha E. Williams and Thomas M. Hogan, comps. Medford, N.J.: Learned Information, Inc., 1981, pp. 29–35.

10. Shirley, Sherrilynne. "A Survey of Computer Search Costs in the Academic Health Sciences Library." *Bulletin of the Medical Library Association* 66 (October 1978):390–6.

11. Boyce, Bert R. "A Cost Accounting Model for Online Computerized Literature Searching." *Journal of Library Administration* 4 (Summer 1983):43–9.

12. Martyn, John, and Lancaster, F. Wilfred. "Cost Analysis." In: Martyn, John and Lancaster, F. Wilfred. *Investigative Methods in Library and Information Science: An Introduction.* Arlingtion, Va.: Information Resources Press, 1981, pp. 175–93.

13. Lynch, Mary Jo. "Libraries Embrace Online Search Fees." *American Libraries* 14 (1982):174.

14. Nielson, Brian. "Teacher or Intermediary: Alternative Professional Models in the Information Age." *College and Research Libraries* 43 (1982):183–91.

15. DesChene, Doris. "An Analysis of Flat Fees for Online Searches." *National Online Meeting Proceedings, 1981,* Martha E. Williams and Thomas M. Hogan, comps. Medford, N.J.: Learned Information, Inc., 1981, pp. 161–5.

Cost Analysis
of a Circuit Library Program

Lillian Levine

ABSTRACT. Circuit library programs are a means of providing library service to small hospitals through the visits of a traveling librarian. The program is administered by a resource library which makes its collections available, hires the librarian, and provides support services. The cost of all the services and materials for the program must be identified. The administering library then determines the method for billing each of the circuit institutions for their share of the costs. The circuit program at the Cleveland Health Sciences Library is described as an example of one method of cost recovery.

INTRODUCTION

Circuit programs have developed in recent years to meet the information needs of small or remote hospitals. These programs provide professional library service which the hospitals might not otherwise be able to afford. They are administered by a resource library which offers service to less developed libraries through a circuit librarian. Administration of the program requires a resource library which can provide a traveling librarian; an adequate collection of books and journals to meet the needs of the participating hospitals; a system for acquiring materials through interlibrary loan; and professional, clerical and administrative personnel to support the librarian. There is a range in the quantity of services offered which depends on the needs of the hospital and the amount of time spent there by the librarian. In any case the librarian

Lillian Levine is Extramural Coordinator and directs the Circuit Library Program at the Cleveland Health Sciences Library of Case Western Reserve University in Cleveland, OH. She has an M.S.L.S. from the School of Library Science of Case Western Reserve University.

would be expected to provide reference services, computer and manual searches, photocopies, and loans. When the librarian is in the hospital more than one or two hours a week, collection development and collection maintenance, including cataloging and serials control would probably be part of the service.

Circuit programs vary in the way they schedule the librarian's time, obtain their funding, bill their participating institutions, and define their services.[1,2,3,4,5] Some programs have been established primarily to bring library service to underserved areas. Others have been initiated to market the services of the resource library. Some circuits include hospitals which are quite close to one another, while others require the librarian to drive as much as 150 miles a day. While some circuit programs are operated from large academic resource libraries, with all their attendant support services, other programs originate from hospital libraries with smaller staffs.

Budgets for circuit programs will vary, therefore, because of the diversity of resources available to hospitals. It is, in fact, important that a careful analysis be made of the hidden or indirect costs, as well as the more apparent direct costs, at the outset of the program. With all expenses considered, the resource institution is less likely to find itself bearing the cost of unanticipated demands made on its staff and budget.

COST ANALYSIS AND COST RECOVERY

The cost analysis of a circuit program can be accomplished in three steps. First, all the possible expenses that could be incurred in the operation of the program for one year are accumulated. Next, it is necessary to determine which items, if any, will be absorbed by the existing operations of the resource library, and which will be charged to the circuit libraries. Finally, the expenses are examined and a method of cost recovery is selected.

Business operating costs are traditionally divided into labor, materials and overhead. It is expected that the resource and circuit libraries would each absorb their own overhead costs. Labor costs include the salaries, fringe benefits and continuing education of the personnel providing library ser-

TABLE I

SERVICES IN A CIRCUIT PROGRAM

Ready Reference	Collection Maintenance
Searches	Statistics and Record Keeping
Collection Development	Photocopying
Cataloging	Billing
Library Committee	Interlibrary Loan (includes
Program Administration	verifying, locating, followup)

TABLE II

MATERIALS FOR A CIRCUIT PROGRAM

On-site collection	Catalog cards
Resource collection	Automobile, gasoline
ALA interlibrary loan forms	Postage and shipping
Terminal for searching	Telephone charges
Connect time	Microcomputer and software
Stationery and supplies	OCLC charges

vice. Personnel may include clerks or assistants as well as the circuit librarian(s) and the program administrator.[2,4] Listed in Table I are the services which may be offered in a circuit program. Some duties are clearly professional, while others may be performed by either the librarian or an assistant. The important thing to remember is that each of these tasks is going to require someone's time and therefore, has some price attached to it.

The second largest part of the program budget is materials. Items which should be considered for the program budget are listed in Table II.

At this point the decision must be made as to which items will be figured into the resource library's operating budget and which will be charged to the circuit libraries. Each library usually pays for its own collection development. The assumption is that the resource library has initiated such a program because of its own substantial collection and will not have to make any major changes in its acquisitions policy. Exceptions may occur, however. An academic institution with excellent holdings in the clinical sciences may discover that it does not have enough materials on hospital administration. The decision must be made as to whether these materials will be purchased or borrowed, and by whom. When a circuit library requests materials from the resource library, will there be a photocopy or loan charge? It may be possible to fit interlibrary loan or billing procedures into already established work-flow routines of the resource library. This will free the circuit librarian's time for other duties. On the other hand, unanticipated expenses may arise. The increased work generated by the circuit program may necessitate hiring an additional assistant or clerk. The personnel policies of the resource institution may require increases in salaries and fringe benefits. It is best to be prepared for all contingencies.

When the expenses have been identified, a method for recovering them can be attempted. An initial consideration is whether the resource library should apply for outside funding. There are some good reasons for considering this option today. If grant money is available, the opportunity to demonstrate to a small hospital the advantages of library service at no cost to the hospital is very appealing. The hospital staff becomes accustomed to its newfound access to medical information, and hopefully the service sells itself. Implicit in this approach is an agreement on the part of the hospital to assume financial responsibility for the library at a later date. A second advantage is the opportunity to evaluate the hospital's use of library services. By keeping careful statistics, one may predict future use, and in that way set fees for the following year. The risk in this approach is that a library's use may not really be predictable. If economic pressures are severe enough, and staff support is not strong, the hospital may decide to cut back on certain library services when they are no longer free.

Once all possible expenses have been accounted for, there are several ways of charging for service. An annual rate may be calculated by totaling the fixed costs: salaries, fringe benefits, continuing education, and travel expenses; and adding to this the estimated cost of materials and time for such variable services as computer searches and interlibrary loan. This method provides all parties involved with a definite amount to write into their budgets.[5] If usage does not meet expectations, however, there may be dissatisfaction on the part of the circuit library, or financial pressure on the resource library. One circuit program's solution is to provide a subscription for a pre-defined amount of service at a fixed price. The hospital then has the option to renew its service as needed.[6]

A second method is to charge a flat rate for those costs likely to remain constant during the year, and a separate per item charge for services whose usage may vary. This insures a basic amount of income to the resource library, and permits some flexibility and control of cost on the part of the circuit library.[2]

Another way to cover costs is to determine an annual rate based on the bed size of the circuit institution. At one Pennsylvania hospital, expenses for the entire circuit program are totaled. This sum is then divided by the number of hospital beds in all the circuit hospitals, thus establishing a per bed charge which can be used to set fees for the coming year.[4]

Another circuit program has modified this system by using a weighted bed ratio to determine fixed costs. An acute care bed is given the value of one, while skilled nursing beds and health-related beds are each counted as a fraction of one. This calculation helps to eliminate disproportionately high costs for the smaller hospitals.[7]

In planning for cost recovery, the resource library must also have some assurance that participating institutions will not unexpectedly drop out of the program. Such an unplanned event leaves the resource library and remaining circuit libraries with the problem of covering that hospital's share of the fixed expenses. Some circuit programs draw up contracts, while others rely on the good faith of the participants in the program.

THE CLEVELAND HEALTH SCIENCES LIBRARY CIRCUIT PROGRAM

The method of cost recovery of the circuit library program at the Cleveland Health Sciences Library (CHSL) of Case Western Reserve University in Cleveland, Ohio, is described here as one way of providing this kind of service. It was started in 1973, and is one of the oldest programs still operating. It is a large program, currently consisting of seven circuit librarians serving twenty-four institutions of varying size and location. Librarians who are examining ways of financing circuit programs may find some of its methods useful, but in the end must base their decisions on the unique characteristics of their own resource and circuit libraries.

The circuit program was initiated at CHSL in response to the requests of hospital administrators who wished to provide library services to their staffs, but could not afford the cost of a full-time or part-time librarian. Many of these hospitals were outside the Greater Cleveland area, and professional librarians were not locally available. Yet there was a pressing need for up-to-date medical information.

The initial circuit was a pilot project to serve five hospitals in two counties east of Greater Cleveland. From the beginning, the program was structured so that each hospital would pay its share of the expenses. There would be no subsidizing of the costs, either by CHSL or by outside funding agencies. This has proven to be a useful policy because it has kept the charges commensurate with the service. Increases and decreases in amount of service have been based on the demonstrated needs of the hospitals and what they have been able to afford.

The success of the first year led to the initiation of two other circuits in 1974. One provided library service to six small hospitals in a rural area south of Cleveland. The second circuit consisted of four small city hospitals within the Greater Cleveland area. By 1977 CHSL was operating seven different circuits. The composition of these circuits has varied over the years, but in general, there have always been three that served city hospitals, three that were more rural in their location, and one or two that served departmental libraries within University Hospitals of Cleveland and the Medical School of Case Western Reserve University. Three of the original hospitals are still circuit participants. During the past eleven years, nine hospitals have experienced library development to the point that they were eventually able to hire a full-time or part-time librarian and maintain their own library independent of the circuit program.

The charging mechanism which was initiated in 1973 is still in effect today. It is based on two factors: a fixed annual charge unique to each circuit, and an itemized fee for specific services which is billed quarterly. The annual charge is derived by listing the fixed costs for each circuit for the coming year. The items which contribute to the fixed charge are: librarian's salary, clerical support, professional support, fringe benefits which are determined by the University, and continuing education for the librarian. The professional support covers a portion of the salary of the administrator of the circuit program. Clerical support from all of the circuits contributes to the salary of one library assistant in CHSL's Interlibrary Loan Department who is responsible for the processing, photocopying, and statistics for billing of all the circuit interlibrary loan transactions. If the librarian's circuit is outside the city, the annual mileage is calculated and reimbursement is added into the fixed annual fee. Automobile and driver's insurance are part of the fixed charges and are figured in with the salary fringe benefits.

The amount of time that the librarian spends at each institution determines the proportion of the total figure that each institution pays. Since the librarian spends one day of each week at CHSL doing reference work and obtaining materials for the entire circuit, each day of service is calculated as one-fourth of the total cost. Therefore, if the fixed costs for a circuit for one year were determined to be $25,600, a library receiving one day per week of service would pay $6,400 per year in fixed charges. The charge for one-half day per week would be $3,200. A sample budget for one circuit is given in Table III.

The variable charges include interlibrary loan and photocopy fees, computerized database searches, and cataloging. The circuit institution provides the library space, equipment, collection materials and supplies. There must be a contact person at the circuit institution willing to take requests during the time that the librarian is not in the hospital. In some of the larger circuit institutions, the hospital provides clerical and/or secretarial assistance for the librarian. Overhead is absorbed by each of the participating institutions.

By itemizing all the anticipated direct costs and presenting

TABLE III

SAMPLE BUDGET

Librarian's Salary	$17,000
Clerical Support	1,470
Professional Support	1,330
Fringe Benefits	4,000
Education	500
Travel	1,300
Total	$25,600

Allocation of charges:

General Hospital	2 days/week	$12,800
Community Hospital	1 day/week	6,400
Memorial Hospital	½ day/week	3,200
Rural Hospital	½ day/week	3,200
Total		$25,600

them to the circuit institution in advance, exorbitant unexpected expenses have been avoided. The circuit institution knows exactly what it is paying for. The cost is proportional to the service provided.

CONCLUSIONS

The kinds of library service offered in a circuit program will be determined by the resources and services of the library providing the service. Similarly, the method of charging will be a reflection of the resource institution, its ability to absorb certain costs, and its mechanisms for bookkeeping and billing. While there is more than one way to balance the budget in a circuit program, three goals should be kept in mind. First of all, no matter what kind of outside funding is originally available, the aim of every program should be, in the end, to be self-supporting. Secondly, some mechanism that permits the charges to reflect actual usage should be built into every fee structure. Finally, institutions in the process of developing circuit programs should be wary of offering more than they can afford to deliver.

REFERENCES

1. Feltovic, Helen F. "Six Coordinated Medical Libraries." *Bulletin of the Medical Library Association* 52 (October 1964):670–75.
2. Feuer, Sylvia. "The Circuit Rider Librarian." *Bulletin of the Medical Library Association* 65 (July 1977):349–53.
3. Gordner, Ronald L. "Riding the Rural Library Circuit." *Medical Reference Services Quarterly* 1 (Spring 1982):59–74.
4. Antes, E. Jean. "A Librarian for the Small Hospital." *Nursing Times* 88 (October 6, 1982):1683–85.
5. Plunket, Linda; Genetti, Raynna Bowlby; Greven, Maryanne Lamont; and Estabrook, Barbara. "Circuit Riding; a Method for Providing Reference Services." *Special Libraries* 74 (January 1983):49–55.
6. Smith, Bernie Todd. Private communication, March 16, 1984.
7. Edsall, Shirley. Private communication, March 19, 1984.

Cost Analysis
of a Document Delivery
Photocopy Service

Gail A. Partin
M. Sandra Wood

ABSTRACT. An analysis of the costs for providing photo-copied articles through an Information Service was performed at the Hershey Medical Center as a tool for decision making and evaluation of the service. The literature written on the cost analysis of document delivery is reviewed and a rationale for cost analysis is provided. Costs are categorized into direct variable costs, direct fixed costs, and indirect costs. The self-observation method was utilized for data collection. Results are presented as unit costs. The decision of what costs to include, both in a cost analysis and a pricing strategy, are dependent on a library's philosophy.

INTRODUCTION

Cost analysis is becoming a more frequently discussed topic within the fields of library and information science. As the emphasis shifts from providing free services to fee-based services, librarians are finding themselves faced with the complex, and sometimes controversial, task of designing a price structure for library services. One of the library services that has traditionally been provided on a fee basis is interlibrary loan, specifically the document delivery of photocopied items.

Gail A. Partin, currently the cataloging clerk, was formerly the manager of the Information Service at the George T. Harrell Library, The Milton S. Hershey Medical Center, The Pennsylvania State University, Hershey, PA 17033. She is also an M.L.S. candidate at Clarion University of Pennsylvania.

M. Sandra Wood is Head, Reference, The George T. Harrell Library, The Milton S. Hershey Medical Center, The Pennsylvania State University, Hershey, PA 17033. She received an M.L.S. from Indiana University and an M.B.A. from the University of Maryland.

As long as technological advancements become available for use in the document delivery function, and as long as networks and cooperative arrangements continue to be restructured, a simple, low cost, reliable approach to cost analysis will be needed. The aim of this paper is to present such an approach and to demonstrate its application to the document delivery of photocopied items. Whether a library elects to charge a fee or provide free service, it must still be aware of what the costs of the service are in order to prepare its budget or engage in the decision-making process.

HISTORICAL BACKGROUND

In 1978 an analysis was made of the Information Service provided to physicians in Pennsylvania by The George T. Harrell Library of The Milton S. Hershey Medical Center. This service had been provided free of charge as part of the Susquehanna Valley Regional Medical Program until 1974, and later was funded from 1974 to 1975 by the Pennsylvania Medical Society. In 1975, when this funding was discontinued, fees were instituted for the Library's Information Service. The authors of that analysis studied the impact of fees and found an initial reduction of one-third in the total number of users of the service, which included both document delivery and brief literature searching.[1] Since that time, physicians' use of the Information Service, specifically document delivery, has remained at a low level. Current usage of the Information Service primarily consists of document delivery to other libraries through various interlibrary loan arrangements.

During most of the 1970s, the Information Service served as an alternative to the Library's participation as a Resource Library in the Regional Medical Library Network, so the Library maintained a dual service with different pricing structures. Until 1982 the National Library of Medicine (NLM) provided full or partial subsidies to libraries requesting document delivery up to a pre-specified quota. When the subsidy was eliminated in 1982, libraries requesting document delivery were required to pay the full cost of $4.50 per item, which was an increase from $2.50 in 1973.

In tandem with the Mid-Eastern Regional Medical Library

Service (MERMLS) fee structure, Harrell Library also maintained a separate Information Service for document delivery supplied to individuals and physicians outside the Medical Center and to other libraries who did not participate in the Regional Medical Library Network. The first fee, imposed in January 1974, was twenty cents per page with a two dollar minimum fee per item photocopied. By July 1979, the fee had increased to $3.50 for any article up to ten pages; additional pages were assessed at twenty-five cents each.

Early in 1983 several changes which profoundly affected the levels and costs of the document delivery service occurred simultaneously. A reconfiguration of the Regional Medical Library Network resulted in the dissolution of MERMLS and the creation of the new Greater Northeastern Regional Medical Library Program, which incorporated former NLM Regions 1, 2 and 3. In conjunction with this reconfiguration, the regional cost of document delivery was increased to six dollars per item. At the same time, based on a variety of internal factors, including staffing level, the Harrell Library decided not to continue in its capacity as a document delivery subcontractor within the new region. This period of transition prompted a reassessment and reevaluation of the Library's Information Service, including costs and price structures for document delivery.

The most immediate consequence of this reassessment was the elimination of the dual price structure that was previously required in order to accommodate the MERMLS subcontract arrangements. Furthermore, the fee charged for document delivery of photocopied items was changed from $3.50 per article up to ten pages photocopied, to $4.50 (billed) per article up to the copyright limit of fifty pages. For articles longer than ten pages, this change resulted in a reduced fee; however, for most items it represented a modest increase.

There also was some evidence that alternative payment methods would be welcomed by both users and staff members alike. For frequent users, a deposit account option, offering a reduced fee of four dollars per item, was developed. This option, currently still available, requires a minimum initial deposit of one hundred dollars. In addition, the Library agreed to accept two different coupons (or stamps) as reimbursement on a per request basis: the College of Physicians of

Philadelphia coupon ($5.00) or the Greater Northeastern Regional Medical Library Coupon ($6.00). The final result, which became effective in January 1983, is a variable fee schedule which permits a user library to choose from a variety of options the payment method that most adequately fits its needs.

During the initial re-evaluation it was recognized that the resolution of several matters would have to be delayed as a consequence of the transition period itself. The Information Service staff felt that the service possessed a significant, but untapped, market potential that could be developed. However, before the market could be expanded, the staff decided initially to take a closer look at the cost analysis and price setting measures employed. For the most part, the fees imposed for the Information Service over the past decade were determined at a rate designed to be competitive with the prevailing regional fees. Ultimately, the decision was made to conduct a cost analysis in 1984, one year after regional reconfiguration, in order to permit the Information Service to stabilize and become more firmly established after undergoing the transition period in early 1983.

LITERATURE REVIEW

A review of library-related literature finds an extremely limited selection of documentation that is pertinent to the cost analysis of information services, and even less information relating to the more specific topic concerning the document delivery of photocopied items. The researcher must wade through a great deal of partially relevant materials in order to ferret out specific bits of appropriate information.

A sizeable portion of this literature addresses the ongoing controversy over "fee-for-service" versus "free" library service. Although it appears to be irrelevant to the specific topic of cost analysis, the concept of "fee" versus "free" must be analyzed and resolved before the benefits of cost analysis can be achieved. Before a fee is implemented, it must strike a precarious balance among several factors: the partial or total recovery of the library's costs, the allowance for flexibility and innovation in the services provided, and the reflection of the library's ability to serve and to practice efficiently within the marketplace.[2]

Much of the cost analysis literature discusses the various elements of price theory, pricing policies, and marketing principles for library functions and services. The marketing concept, a key idea in modern marketing techniques, centers around user needs and consumer satisfaction rather than around the internal organizational structure. Based on this user-oriented concept, a strategy, or "marketing mix," must be formulated which satisfactorily blends the factors of product, place of distribution, price, and promotion.[3,4] As an integral part of the "marketing mix," price strategy can be developed according to a plethora of methods and theories.[5,6]

The cost analysis of library functions is another large component of relevant literature. However, much of the recent information centers around general concepts, overviews, or specific, detailed analysis of library functions such as online database searching.[6,7] These articles, while numerous and informative, can serve only as sources for the most basic guidelines in the cost analysis of document delivery services.

A small fraction of the cost analysis literature actually discusses conducting an evaluation of the document delivery of photocopied items. In the late 1960s and early 1970s, several reports and studies were undertaken to substantiate cost figures. A few articles break the document delivery function down into lists of individual operations or tasks normally performed, and then discuss the costs associated with each task.[8,9] Others are indepth reports of the various methods utilized for interlibrary loan cost studies.

The most definitive and often quoted interlibrary loan cost study was conducted by Vernon Palmour and others for the Association of Research Libraries.[10] Published in 1972, it appears to be the most recent nationwide study of academic interlibrary loan costs that can be found in the literature. This study had several purposes, one of which was to determine the average cost per interlibrary loan transaction. Cost data were obtained from twelve large academic libraries and thirteen associated branches. These data were then compiled to yield separate cost figures for borrowing and lending, each of which were further subdivided to determine the individual costs for filled or unfilled requests. Based on direct costs and a fifty percent overhead, the average lending cost per request was $2.12 for an unfilled loan request and $4.67 for a filled loan request. Interestingly, there was a rather wide range of costs among the twelve large libraries participating—from a high of $6.81 to a low of $2.05 for a filled loan request. No significant correlation could be made between cost per transaction and collection size. However, the study did acknowledge that geographical location, proportion of professional staffing, degree of centralization, and efficiency of the unit may have accounted for the wide variation in costs among the libraries studied. The ultimate aim of the study was to collect "valid cost data that can be used for planning at both the national and local level."[10]

More recently, an interlibrary loan cost study was undertaken at the University of Oklahoma in 1978.[11] Although conducted only as an internal cost analysis device, the study provides much relevant information in its methodology, as well as in its comparisons to the Palmour study. Especially pertinent is the example set by this study: that sound cost data can be obtained without implementing additional staff or slowing down the workflow, that data can be compiled manually without the necessity of computers, and that results can be analyzed and evaluated by personnel who are not trained statisticians.

A unique cost study conducted prior to the Palmour study was reported in 1971 by Carol Spencer of the College of Physicians of Philadelphia.[12] Unit costs of providing interlibrary loans and photocopies were determined by random time sampling and self-observation. Personnel costs were measured by logging working time on a checklist of tasks at randomly chosen intervals. All staff members involved in the study were issued a Random Alarm Mechanism (RAM) which, when activated, signalled the worker to record the appropriate tasks being performed at that time. This study was especially helpful in its enumeration of the multitude of separate tasks and cost units which comprise each interlibrary lending transaction.

For the most part, the costs per transaction of these interlibrary loan studies have purposefully been excluded from the preceding discussion for several reasons. First, all of these studies were conducted prior to 1980; hence, the results which were reported in the form of dollar amounts must be considered out of date. Also, no two studies were conducted in a similar enough manner to be validly compared. Even after careful analysis of all the methodologies, the results of these studies still can be only loosely compared because of the myriad complexities of the data collection and compilation procedures utilized. This is because diverse internal practices and procedures have prevented libraries from adopting one standard method for determining the costs of library functions.

METHODOLOGY

The first step taken by the Harrell Library, even before deciding upon the data collection method, was to determine and categorize all of the costs involved in its document delivery service. All costs were broken down into the following three categories:[6]

1. Direct Variable Costs. These are costs that relate to each use of the document delivery service and that include such things as supplies, specified personnel costs, communications use, photocopying expenses and postage.
2. Direct Fixed Costs. These costs are incurred only one time, whether or not any use takes place. Examples include the costs associated with maintenance of the collection, including acquisition, binding, storage, and weeding.
3. Indirect Costs. This includes those costs which are not affected by the amount of usage. Examples include overhead items, rent, and administration.

This first step of assigning categories to each cost unit was probably the most important task in terms of facilitating the manipulation and understanding of the final data. It was also the most confusing, and required a great deal of indepth study because of the variety of options for classification available. These three categories were chosen by the Harrell Library because they most clearly define the relationship between total cost and "number of uses." For the most part, the variable cost per unit remains fairly constant over a range of "number of uses." However, when the fixed or the indirect costs are added, the average unit cost per use decreases as the total number of uses increases. Therefore, the proportion of fixed and indirect costs is greatest for a small number of uses. When costs are calculated separately for each of these categories, new insight can be gained into the interrelationships of the various library functions and services.

A variety of methods can be implemented for the data collection phase of a cost study. An often-used method for determining costs is to retrospectively gather data on an annual, semi-annual, or quarterly basis. The central premise for this approach is that costs are estimated for the time period decided upon. All three cost categories are determined by estimation. Using this method, fixed and indirect costs are calculated in many studies as percentages of direct wages. The exact percentage is determined within each institution depending upon its definition of the costs included in each category. Although there are widespread interpretations of fixed and indirect costs as well as the percentages utilized, it is a common practice to estimate these categories in the manner described. To do otherwise would require very time-consuming, complicated accounting procedures that could be justified in only the largest libraries.

Variable costs (such as supplies, labor, equipment, and postage) present a more complicated picture. Depending upon the accounting procedures employed, it may be impossible to make an accurate estimate of the supplies and postage consumed by only a small section of the library. Additionally, separate costs for equipment and communication expenses may be unobtainable. Labor costs can be more easily estimated but may not be any more accurate than the other estimates. Each employee involved in any phase of the interlibrary loan photocopy service is identified. A determination of the percentage of total work time spent on document delivery tasks is then made for each employee. This estimate can be made by the employer and/or the supervisor. The employee's annual salary, including fringe benefits, is then multiplied by the appropriate percentage of time spent on document delivery tasks. All of these costs are combined to provide the total variable cost for the time period under study.

Another approach to data collection is the work sampling

method.[12] For the time periods designated, each employee engaged in those document delivery operations being studied completes a log sheet indicating the number of minutes spent working on each task. The amount of time each employee spends working on specified tasks can then be totaled and equated with the appropriate hourly wage. When each employee's labor costs, including fringe benefits, are calculated and totaled, an accurate figure for personnel costs is obtained. The log sheet completed by each employee is the key to this approach because it can also be used to record the exact amount and type of materials consumed, as well as to record the number and disposition of each transaction discharged by the unit. This self-observation, work-sampling technique, permits a degree of indepth analysis that is not otherwise achieved by the estimation method. As in the estimation method, fixed and indirect costs for the work sampling method are calculated as a percentage of direct wages.

The University of Oklahoma study done in 1978 used the estimation approach to determine labor costs, but also used a ledger sheet approach for collecting data concerning the other variable costs. Spencer, though, adhered strictly to the self-observation, work-sampling approach in her study conducted at the College of Physicians of Philadelphia, and found it to be a low cost, reliable way to obtain indepth cost data without undue interference in normal department operations.[12] By contrast, the Palmour study employed variations in both of these methods to determine variable costs. He found that the best overall estimate of labor costs was provided by estimating the number of hours each employee spent engaged in interlibrary loan activities. According to Palmour, "the logging of time spent on individual tasks always leads to an underestimate of the actual time."[10,11]

For several reasons, the Harrell Library chose to collect data according to the basic work-sampling approach. Unlike many high volume document delivery services, the Harrell Library does not divide its photoduplication service into a separate, distinct department. Therefore, employees working in document delivery at the Library also are expected to perform other duties which are not part of the photocopy service. This means that all of the labor costs are variable because no employee spends one hundred percent of his or her time engaged in document delivery activities. Also, there is no internal accounting procedure to determine the amount of supplies and postage used for document delivery purposes only because these amounts are charged to the budget according to library-wide consumption. Therefore, the only way for the Library to determine an accurate figure for labor, supplies and postage was to keep a log sheet which recorded these costs as they were incurred.

DATA COLLECTION

A random, self-observation technique was chosen in order to gather an accurate sampling of the work. To minimize the amount of distortion that is created by the collection process itself, a ten-day time period was selected as adequate for a representative sample. To provide randomness and to avoid the effects of peak periods and other atypical distortions, the ten survey days were spread over a seven-week period by selecting every fourth working day as a survey day.

Since data were to be collected on a daily basis, a Daily Data Collection Sheet was designed to coordinate with the existing daily routines. Each employee completed only those sections relating to the tasks performed for the day. The data sheet provided space to record the following tasks or items:

1. Date.
2. Number of Transactions. This included filled and unfilled photocopy requests which were completed on the survey day.
3. Activities. The actual start and stop times were recorded for the five activities listed below. Included in these times were rest periods, personal breaks, and other interruptions relating to the lending operation, such as answering or asking questions and taking telephone calls.

    a. Receiving Requests
       —Opening mail
       —Taking phone requests
       —Checking TWX machine

—Checking OCLC pending file and printing
out each request
—Date stamping and sorting requests
—Verifying title and/or citation
—Determining ownership/availability
—Searching for item and pulling from shelves
b. Photocopying
—Sign out auditron for copying machine
—Copy pages requested
—Count pages and mark on request form
—Stamp each request with copyright notice
—Arrange in groups by requester name
c. Billing/Charging
—Determine requester's chosen payment
method
—Prepare invoice or statement of account
—Maintain record of all accounts
—Post invoices and statements
—Follow up overdue invoices and notices
—Record all transactions in logbook for statis-
tics
d. Sending requests
—Prepare proper sized envelope
—Reply via TWX or OCLC
—Reshelving
e. Resolving problem requests

4. Photocopier use. This included three separate tabula-
tions.

a. Article length. The number of pages copied per
transaction was recorded.
b. Copier paper used. This was the number of sheets
of photocopier paper used, and was simply a count
of the sheets of paper used in the machine. It was
always different from article length because two-
sided copying was done.
c. Copier exposure. This count was taken from a me-
ter located inside the copy machine. This was necessary because the copiers were rented, and the
Library was charged a rental/maintenance fee per
exposure.

5. Postage costs. For survey days, document delivery mail was kept separate from other Library mail and taken to the inhouse post office for tabulation of postal charges.
6. Supplies. The various sized envelopes, labels, form letters, etc., were listed and an indication was made each time an item was used. Supplies discarded due to errors also were counted because mistakes are a normal cost of providing service.

As soon as the Daily Data Collection Sheet was designed and reproduced, Information Service staff members were given a copy to review. Recording procedures were discussed with special emphasis given to timekeeping for the five activities. Each activity was defined to include the tasks as listed above. However, time was recorded according to the five primary activities only, not by each individual task listed. Prior to the start of the study, document delivery staff were provided with a list of the ten days on which the study was to be conducted, in order to avoid confusion. The final step was to execute a one day trial run of the collection process so that unanticipated problems could be resolved.

RESULTS

Before the study was undertaken, a simple test to ensure adequate sample size was devised. The average number of pages (article length) per transaction was calculated for the preceding twelve-month period by using the Library's own internal statistics. The annual average was 8.69 pages per transaction. If the average article, the time period would have to be extended in order to increase the sample size so that a similar average would result. Therefore, the first calculation performed at the conclusion of the ten-day study was to determine the average number of pages per transaction. The result was 8.66 pages per transaction; thus, the sample size was found to be valid.

The information recorded on the ten daily log sheets was compiled into a single set of data so that costs could be calculated. Personnel costs were determined by totaling the number of hours each employee spent engaged in the activities enumerated. The proper hourly wage was allotted for each employee. Fringe benefits, calculated at 31.6 percent of hourly wages, were then added. This figure was supplied by the institution's grant department and is considered to be a standard rate for the entire facility. The total cost of direct labor was divided by the total number of transactions to acquire a labor unit cost of $1.62 per item.

Photocopier use was determined by multiplying the cost per exposure by the total number of exposures. Based on the Library's lease agreement, a cost of four cents was assessed per exposure. This amount included the costs of machine rental, maintenance, toner, and developing fluid. The unit cost for paper, envelopes, and other supplies was calculated according to the latest invoice amounts available. The total cost for each item was obtained by multiplying the unit cost by the number of supply items used. These figures were combined and then divided by the total number of transactions to provide a per item cost of $.38 for supplies and equipment. Postage costs also were calculated in the same fashion, and were determined to be $.22 per transaction.

By adding the unit cost figures for direct labor, photocopier use, supplies, equipment, and postage, the variable cost per transaction can be ascertained. In this study the variable cost was determined to be $2.22 per item. It should be pointed out that no communications costs were included in this figure since the document delivery section did not incur any direct charges for telephone, TWX or OCLC during the course of the study, although these costs do occur on an annual basis. There are never any variable expenses resulting from the use of OCLC for document delivery because the fee for using the ILL subsystem is imposed upon the borrowing, not the lending library. The telephone and TWX machine are similar to the OCLC terminal in that the expense is assessed to the library that initiates the transaction. Virtually all replies are made via U.S. mail, either by sending a photocopy of the item or by mailing an unfilled request form. Since telephone and TWX communications for the Information Service are negligible, fixed costs for these services were not included in this study.

Indirect costs, or overhead, were estimated as a percentage of the total direct wages, then broken down into an average cost per request which could be compared to or combined with the variable unit cost. The overhead cost was calculated at 60 percent with an additional administrative cost assessed at ten percent. The overhead unit cost was $.74 and included expenses for general institutional level administration, personnel services, rental of office space, depreciation of building and equipment, housekeeping, and general maintenance. The administrative unit cost, assessed at $.12 per request, included library administration, supervision and training of document delivery staff, formulation of policies and procedures for the service, and a share of the expenses associated with membership in cooperative interlibrary loan networks such as OCLC and the Regional Medical Library Network. The indirect unit cost was determined to be $.86 per request, which was ascertained by combining the overhead and administrative unit costs.

It may be appropriate to digress at this point and compare fringe benefit and overhead percentages as determined over the past decade. In 1971, Carol Spencer calculated fringe benefits at ten percent of direct wages, and overhead at 45 percent of direct wages.[12] Her definition of overhead was comparable to overhead plus administrative costs given in this report. In 1972, Palmour used 15 percent for fringe benefits and 50 percent for overhead, both calculated as percentage of direct wages and defined similarly to Spencer's report.[10] In 1981 the University of Oklahoma conducted its cost analysis using Palmour's overhead and fringe benefit rates. This was done primarily to facilitate the comparison of results between the Palmour study, conducted on a national level, and the University of Oklahoma's cost analysis, conducted solely as an internal measurement. Within the Harrell Library, fringe benefits have steadily increased from 12 percent in 1975, to 20 percent in 1979, to 31.6 percent in 1984; and overhead costs have ranged from 45 percent to 57 percent over the past decade. The addition of a ten percent administrative cost factor to the indirect cost category also appears to be appropriate. In *Cost Analysis of Library Functions,* Mitchell, Tanis and Jaffe strongly advocate including the administrative function in any study of cost factors. Also, they revealed "the somewhat startling fact that 36 percent of . . . total labor hours and 44 percent of total labor costs are attributable to non-unit-producing functions such as Administration, Training, Personnel, Administrative Support, Miscellaneous (e.g., vacation, sick leave, coffee breaks), and other functions such as Systems Analysis and Programming."[7]

Since 1983 the document delivery service has undergone several major personnel changes, thus requiring above normal amounts of training and supervision. Also requiring abnormally high training time as well as the reorganization of workflow, procedures, and department policies was the acquisition of an OCLC terminal and membership into OCLC's Interlibrary Loan Subsystem. Since the close of this study period, the service has acquired a telefacsimile machine and is currently participating in a cooperative network, with the capacity to provide full text document delivery within one hour from receipt of a request. Future trends such as telefacsimile networks, electronic mail, and full text data transmission will irrevocably change the nature of document delivery services. Both changes in staffing and advancements in technology result in real administrative costs which must be reflected in the cost study.

The final cost category, direct fixed costs, was defined for this study as the costs of acquisition and maintenance of the collection. Both Palmour and Spencer agree that there are real costs involved with acquiring and maintaining the collection and that some of these costs should be allocated to the document delivery service since it is a primary user of the collection. Although previous cost analysis studies have not routinely included collection costs, the Palmour study does provide several approaches to the subject; and Spencer warns that these fixed costs could easily exceed the variable or indirect costs.

The approach used in this study was to determine the proportion of collection costs to be applied to the Information Service. The following formula was employed:

$$\frac{\text{Number of ILL Lending Transactions}}{\text{(Total Circulation} + \text{(Number of ILL Lending Transactions)}} \times \text{Collection Costs} =$$

Amount to be applied to the Information Service

TABLE 1

DOCUMENT DELIVERY UNIT COSTS

	Unit Cost(s)	Cumulative Unit Cost ($)
Direct Variable Costs		
Wages	1.23	
Fringe (31.6%)	.39	1.62
Supplies and Equipment	.38	2.00
Postage	.22	2.22
Indirect Costs		
Overhead (60%)	.74	2.96
Administrative (10%)	.12	3.08
Direct Fixed Costs		
Collection Cost	2.14	5.22

This resulted in 3.37 percent of the collection costs, or $8,925.00, being distributed over the annual number of lending transactions. Collection cost elements can include such expenses as acquisition, cataloging, check-in, claiming, marking, binding, storage, shelf-maintenance and depreciation. For this study only acquisition and binding costs were included because these figures were readily available and required no special expertise to ascertain. The final unit cost for fixed costs was determined to be $2.14 per lending transaction. Perhaps it was not deemed especially important in 1971 and 1972 to include collection costs. However, in view of steadily increasing subscription prices, it may be totally unrealistic in 1984 to exclude such expenses from the document delivery cost analysis process.

The final cost figures are presented in Table 1. Results are presented as unit costs, with a cumulative unit cost figure.

CONCLUSION

Different approaches may be taken for implementing a cost analysis study depending upon the type of function being analyzed, the staffing levels available to conduct the study, and the library's philosophy toward reimbursement for services rendered. Each library must evaluate its own market potential as well as all of the various options before making a final decision on pricing strategy. Two popular options are full cost recovery or partial cost recovery of expenses incurred. Another option is differential pricing designed to encourage or discourage certain types of users. Still other options include price setting for profits or competitive pricing.

Regardless of the price structure used, every library needs to secure some method for accumulating relevant data for planning and decision making. This report describes one method which can be successfully implemented in an efficient, cost-effective manner by personnel without specialized training in statistics. The results can provide a basis for comparison with other internal library functions and other libraries, or simply provide a useful tool for evaluating and planning library functions.

REFERENCES

1. Lehman, Lois J., and Wood, M. Sandra. "Effect of Fees on an Information Service for Physicians." *Bulletin of the Medical Library Association* 66 (January 1978):58–61.

2. Cheshier, Robert G. "Fees for Service in Medical Library Networks." *Bulletin of the Medical Library Association* 60 (April 1972):325–32.

3. Edinger, Joyce A. "Marketing Library Services: Strategy for Survival." *College and Resource Libraries* 41 (July 1980):328–32.

4. Shapiro, Stanley J. "Marketing and the Information Professional." *Special Libraries* 71 (November 1980):409–14.

5. Kibirige, Harry M. *The Information Dilemma: A Critical Analysis of Information Pricing and the Fees Controversy.* Westport, Conn.: Greenwood Press, 1983.

6. King, Donald W. "Pricing Policies in Academic Libraries." *Library Trends* 28 (Summer 1979):47–62.

7. Mitchell, Betty Jo; Tanis, Norman E.; Jaffe, Jack. *Cost Analysis of Library Functions.* Greenwich, Conn.: Jai Press, 1978.

8. Phelps, Ralph H. "Factors Affecting the Costs of Library Photocopying." *Special Libraries* 58 (February 1967):113.

9. Sullivan, Robert C. "Report of the Photocopying Costs in Libraries Committee." *Library Resources and Technical Services* 14 (Spring 1970):279–89.

10. *A Study of the Characteristics, Costs, and Magnitude of Interlibrary Loans in Academic Libraries,* comp. by Vernon E. Palmour and others, prepared for the Association of Research Libraries by Westat Research, Inc. Westport, Conn.: Greenwich Press, 1972.

11. Herstand, Jo Ellen. "Interlibrary Loan Cost Study and Comparison." *RQ* 20 (Spring 1981):249–56.

12. Spencer, Carol C. "Random Time Sampling with Self-Observation for Library Cost Studies: Unit Costs of Interlibrary Loans and Photocopies at a Regional Medical Library." *Journal of the American Society for Information Science* 22 (May-June 1971):153–60.

II. COST RECOVERY FOR REFERENCE SERVICES

One use for cost analysis is to facilitate pricing decisions. A frequent pricing strategy used by libraries is cost recovery, where a library decides to recover full or partial costs for services. Arcari reviews cost recovery of library services with an emphasis on academic health sciences libraries. The article on the MEDLAR's pricing algorithm by Tilley and Kenton describes the rationale used by the National Library of Medicine in determining its new pricing structure. Caldwell, Mann and Barnard discuss the change in a library's pricing structure for online search services, based on NLM's new algorithm. The hospital library must retool financially in a changing society; Bastille presents the idea of an "entrepreneurial" hospital library. Arcari takes a final look at cost recovery by analyzing funding for a clinical librarian program.

An Overview of Cost Recovery

Ralph D. Arcari

ABSTRACT. Academic health center libraries appear to have developed fee schedules for their services as a matter of routine. Unlike their public or university library counterparts, serious reservations regarding fee for services do not seem to be part of the medical library literature. This paper will discuss cost recovery library services with a specific emphasis on academic health sciences libraries; the University of Connecticut Health Center Library will serve as an example of one such library.

BACKGROUND

The subject heading in *Library Literature* under which one may locate articles on cost recovery is "Fees for Library Services." This heading did not appear until 1972. Before that time articles on library fees were associated with those on fines. Overdue notices, delinquent borrowers and fine forgiveness are the subjects for the majority of articles on library fines and fees until the early 1970s. At that time the issue of charging library patrons for services received its own identity in *Library Literature*. The different orientation of public libraries and medical libraries can be seen in the first articles under "Fees for Library Service" in the years 1972 and 1973.

Barbara Tuchman, the popular historian, suggested in the *New York Times Book Review* that the New York Public Library consider coin-operated turnstiles as a means of generating needed operating revenue to forestall further deterioration of the library.[1] The New York Public Library subsequently rejected the turnstile proposal as impractical.[2]

At the same time, Robert Cheshier's article, "Fees for Ser-

Ralph D. Arcari is the Director of the University of Connecticut Health Center Library, Farmington, CT 06032. He received his M.L.S. from Drexel University in Philadelphia.

vice in Medical Library Networks," was published in the *Bulletin of the Medical Library Association*.[3] Cheshier described the Cleveland Health Science Library cooperative through which dues paying members receive a package of medical library services, including interlibrary loan. In 1973, the National Library of Medicine announced its charges for MEDLINE services.[4] The rates were to be $6.00 per connect hour and $0.10 per offprint page.

The professional literature for the past ten years is replete with articles which question whether public or academic libraries should charge for services. Medical library literature, on the other hand, is more concerned with cost analysis to determine how much one should charge. University and public libraries have been debating the public policy and economic considerations of the impact user charges will make on information access. Health sciences libraries have concentrated on cost determination and allocation. Interlibrary loan is one area, however, where all libraries appear reluctant to assume full service costs. Charges for computer-assisted literature searches have divided the library community.

PUBLICLY SUPPORTED LIBRARIES

The opposition to library fees as public policy was stated by John Berry in an editorial in *Library Journal* entitled "Double Taxation."

> To abandon the tradition [of free public education] and turn our public institutions into the kind of informational and recreational supermarkets suggested by fee enthusiasts is to junk a fundamental right to education and information and to abandon the information need of that part of society that can least afford the price.[5]

Expanding on Berry's concerns, Fay M. Blake and Edith L. Perlmutter took an adamant position against user fees in any publicly supported library. In their "Rush to User Fees," the authors state that:

> Publicly funded libraries and information agencies, however, should guard fiercely against the installation of fees

for services, should provide for services out of rationally planned and expanded budgets, should purchase services from the private sector circumspectly, and at competitive prices.[6]

For Blake and Perlmutter the cost in deprivation of information to the student, faculty member or community person which fees create, far outweighs any benefit to the library. Federal taxation of the private sector should fund public sector information service.

A variation on the Blake and Perlmutter proposal is that of the information stamp or coupon. The latter would be provided to the information indigent through a distribution system similar to that for food stamps.[7] Such a system would allow fees to be imposed without creating any economic barriers to access.

Complete assumption of online search costs in a library's budget has been done at California State College Stanislaus. Paula J. Crawford and Judith A. Thompson report that as a low profile, unadvertized service, no charge online searching is absorbed within the library's operating budget.[8] This method, of course, eliminates the financial barrier issue and allows the library to cancel printed indexes without feeling that such cancellations penalize those who cannot pay.

Libraries are not readily assuming the costs, however, for fees associated with computer searching. John Linford noted in his article, "To Charge or not to Charge," a rationale that "there is a line somewhere where the patron takes over the responsibility of the search."[9] The location of this line has been the subject of economic evaluations of the library fee-for-service question. In two articles in *Library Journal* in 1979, Marilyn Killebrew Gill takes a middle ground on user fees. She states that:

> Use of user fees to finance select services will lead neither to the salvation of the public library nor to its demise. Public pricing is an economically viable, socially sound way to expand some services and improve others. It should be used, however, only to supplement support from general tax revenue, not to supplant it.[10]

Donald W. King in his economic analysis of library fees took a position similar to that in Gill's articles. He concluded that whether or not charges should be made for library services "depend(s) on the type of materials or services involved, their externalities, the type of uses, the cost of materials or services and the cost of administering charges."[11] Externalities is a specific economic term that relates to indirect benefits that are less easily quantifiable than direct costs. The cultural value of a library to its community would be an externality. In short, Gill and King see library fees as an economic judgement dependent on a number of contingencies.

From the revulsion expressed by Blake and Perlmutter to the economic ratiocinations of Gill and Drake, library fees now seem to be relatively accepted through acquiescence and necessity in public institutions. Miriam Drake, in her review of the fee-for-service issue arrives at this point by stating:

> Many public libraries will depend upon a combination of fees and tax funding. . . .We are all concerned with the survival of public libraries and continuance of taxpayer support for services benefitting society, children, students, and the disadvantaged. In order to achieve our goals, we may have to compromise our ideals.[12]

INTERLIBRARY LOANS

As noted above, interlibrary loan is one service in which academic and medical libraries have shown equal interest in cost recovery. Studies have determined costs that either may be assumed by the borrowing institution, passed on to the requesting individual, or reimbursed by a government program.[13,14] As the latter has decreased in practice and costs have risen, more institutions are charging. "The proportion of research libraries that charge fees for interlibrary loans has more than doubled in six years, from 15 percent in 1976 to 33 percent in 1982."[15] The rationale for charging for interlibrary loans may be seen as an institutional financial self-defense. Libraries have limited funds; one clear place to draw the fee-for-service line that Linford referred to is with individuals who have no direct affiliation with the library. Interlibrary loans easily fall into this category.

HEALTH SCIENCES LIBRARIES

While many libraries show little resistance in charging for interlibrary loans, academic health centers often offer a full range of services that are fee-based. The publications of medical librarians reflect this tendency to charge for services. Claire Schultz, formerly Director of the Moore Library of Medicine, Medical College of Pennsylvania, described the methods that one can use to make the library a cost center within its institution.[16] Richard Lyders, Director of the Library of the Houston Academy of Medicine–Texas Medical Center has reported on the system and procedures his library administration has taken to allocate costs proportionally to the users of his library.[17] Paul B. Kantor, a management consultant working under the support of a grant from the National Library of Medicine, recently published his report on the costs of providing health sciences library service.[18] Kantor sampled 24,000 use responses and determined by working with libraries in Cleveland, Los Angeles and Houston the costs to circulate a book ($5.30), to answer a single reference query ($12.63), and to provide space and materials for one hour of study ($8.29).

Carol Spencer used a random sampling technique to determine the costs of various types of reference questions at the National Library of Medicine.[19] One step direction queries, for example, were determined to cost $.044 based on time and salary.

In her analysis of reference costs to individuals not associated with the Library of the University of Oregon Health Sciences Center, Leslie Cable found that such costs averaged $5.18.[20] This cost determination effort was made as part of the research to establish fees for members and non-members in the Oregon Health Information Network.

A review of the medical library literature on cost recovery shows little disinclination on the part of medical libraries to charge for services. There are four factors that may explain the difference between medical librarians and university and public librarians in their respective responses to fees for services. These are the National Library of Medicine, the National Institutes of Health and other granting agencies, the financial structure of academic health centers, and third party payers.

National Library of Medicine

The National Library of Medicine (NLM) plays a significant role in the formation of medical library policies and programs. This is understandable because NLM is the only Federally-supported library providing programs, funding and planning on a national level to effect information transfer to those considered its constituency, i.e., health professionals. The National Library of Medicine has been charging users for access to its databases—MEDLINE, CATLINE, TOXLINE and others—for over a decade. Academic medical libraries, consequently, are familiar with receiving charges from a library providing a service that is part of their daily operations. To model their own fee structure after that of NLM would be consistent with the experience of health sciences libraries.

The Biomedical Communications Network (BCN) is an NLM-sponsored hierarchical structure designed to facilitate document delivery and interlibrary loans. The four levels in this system are:

A. Basic Health Sciences Libraries, usually hospital libraries.
B. Resource or Academic Health Center Libraries.
C. Regional Medical Libraries under contract with NLM for a specific geographic region in the U.S. of which there are now seven.
D. The National Library of Medicine.

Requests for books, journal articles and audiovisuals are directed upward through this network. Initially, NLM reimbursed the provider libraries, while the borrowing libraries received materials at no cost to themselves. Reimbursement was gradually phased out between 1979 and 1982 so that the network is on a complete cost recovery basis now. The experience of medical libraries in making the transition from a free to a fee system under the policy directives of a national library substantially assisted in the formation of medical library cost recovery policies at the regional and local level. As part of the BCN experience, Regional Medical Libraries and Resource Libraries not only were asked to develop and implement fee schedules but also to complete regular cost analyses developed at NLM to determine how much a filled request, a referral or a rejection actually cost. Health sciences libraries, consequently, were required to evaluate their operations in terms of charges to users and justification for those charges. Medical libraries alone in the United States have received this type of national direction. Their participation in the BCN is probably the most significant factor that explains the difference between health sciences libraries and public or university libraries on the issue of user fees.

National Institutes of Health and Granting Agencies

Academic health centers are the nation's research institutions for biomedicine in conjunction with the National Institutes of Health (NIH). The grants awarded to medical and dental schools to further the congressionally-mandated research responsibilities of NIH have both direct and indirect costs associated with them. The direct costs cover actual program expenses, e.g., personnel, equipment and operating costs. Indirect costs include heating, lighting, and support services. The health sciences library along with the personnel, purchasing and accounting departments is a support service for indirect cost calculations.

Academic health center libraries frequently are asked to assist in the determination of costs that can be included in the institutional formula negotiated with NIH for indirect cost reimbursement. Academic health center libraries understand that their institutions are recieving funds that cover the library as an indirect cost. Moreover, federal and private grants can include library photocopying, interlibrary loan and computer search charges as direct costs. Consequently, there is relatively little compunction on the part of the library director to establish fee schedules for faculty members who have access to grant support.

Academic Health Center Financial Structures

The cost center concept is fundamental to the academic health center financial structure. Internal services are on a fee basis, with each major department charging for its services. Physical plant may charge for relocation of furniture or the installation of a floodlight, while Data Services has a fee schedule for the use of the Center's computer and A/V productions charges for developing photographs, graphics and videotape recording. In this environment library charges are a norm rather than an exception as would be the case in public libraries. An academic health center has multiple sources of income: public support, private grants, research grants, tuition funds, hospital fees and outpatient clinic income. Here departments are encouraged to operate on a self-sufficiency basis. The budget officer will encourage fee schedules, cash flow projections and interdepartmental charging.

Smaller hospital libraries often have not implemented cost centers to the extent found in academic health centers. A hospital library may be given an annual amount for photocopying or computer searching to be used, within certain limits, for all hospital departments. In a hospital it may be more efficient for the budget officer to provide one hospital photocopy account to the library rather than allocating separate small sums for this purpose to each department.

Accounts Receivable Department and Third Party Payers

Academic health centers are usually associated with a patient care facility which is accustomed to high volume billing of insurance companies and group health plans for services rendered. An institutional accounts receivable department often handles this function and is responsible for posting funds received to their proper account. Academic health center libraries may have their billing done through accounts receivable and monitor their account balances through monthly income/expenditure statements. The academic health center library is, therefore, one department in an institution with multiple departments, each of which bills for services. Academic health centers provide the support structures that allow a library to charge fees as part of a larger operational pattern.

UNIVERSITY OF CONNECTICUT
HEALTH CENTER LIBRARY

The University of Connecticut Health Center (UCHC) Library is typical of an academic health center library in that it has had the experience of association with NLM policies and has the features of an academic health center department. Fees for services, along with cost recovery analyses, are routine at the UCHC Library.

Interlibrary loan requests are filled according to the guidelines and procedures of the Regional Medical Library (RML) for Region 1 in which UCHC is located. Requests must be accompanied by a prepaid $6.00 RML coupon which UCHC redeems on a monthly basis through the RML. Photocopying may be done by in house users on a coin operated machine; the Library also sells vendacards that will activate a photocopier and eliminate a patron's need for change. Library photocopying for UCHC faculty and staff is $3.00 per article; a similar service for those not associated with UCHC is $6.00/ article. Computer-assisted literature searching is provided at $10.00 per search over the direct online charge from the database vendor. The UCHC fees are based primarily on the following factors:

1. The Library will provide a no cost alternative to those services for which there is a charge. Therefore, a patron may use *Index Medicus* at no charge or request a MEDLINE search for which there is a fee. Clearly, as the costs of indexes increase and the costs to search online decrease relatively, there will be a strong economic impetus for the Library to use the funds for index acquisitions to provide computer access to equivalent databases. The UCHC Library is now only charging where a patron request for a service has caused the Library to incur charges from a vendor—either a photocopy supplier, database service or delivery service for interlibrary loans.

2. Library personnel costs are not included in database search fees because the librarians performing the searches would be employed even if UCHC did not have the capability to do computer-assisted literature searching. Without a computer searching ability, manual searching would be performed. Included in the UCHC charge for searches are continuing education costs for travel to workshops, expenses for manuals and directories, and depreciation on equipment. Library personnel costs are included in the determination of

photocopy and interlibrary loan charges. Personnel in the photocopy and interlibrary loan department are paid from the income generated by this service. Photocopying and interlibrary loan are seen as services for which the Library has received no institutional support funds.

3. Cost analyses are regularly conducted to determine if the Library fees are covering costs. These analyses usually involve sampling the work flow through a department for a specific period of time and associating salary costs with the amount of time spent on individual functions.

4. All fees collected are cash or payment in advance, if possible. Billing is limited to institutional transactions when repayment is not possible. Any patron may charge services against Visa or Mastercharge.

The Library, like other departments at UCHC, can retain its income in a revolving account. This money does not revert to a general fund nor does it lapse at the end of the year. This arrangement is a strong inducement to be cost effective. The revolving account must, however, be budgeted annually, showing all anticipated expenses and identifying cash flow on a quarterly basis. Moreover, all UCHC revolving fund accounts must have a "fall back" account that can be debited should a negative balance occur in the primary account.

CONCLUSION AND FUTURE PERSPECTIVE

Academic health center libraries are more inclined to charge for services than public or university libraries because of their experience with the National Library of Medicine, their administrative environment and their institutional budgetary structures. The University of Connecticut Health Center Library is typical of academic health center libraries in its approach to fees for service.

Given the financial realities of the 1980s, a large federal deficit, decreased funds for social services, and more emphasis on self-supporting service programs, it is probable that university and public libraries will assume operational policies more similar to that of academic health sciences libraries.

REFERENCES

1. Tuchman, Barbara W. "Turnstiles in the Library?" *New York Times Book Review* (March 26, 1972): 2,10.

2. "NYPL Shelves Turnstile Plan as Impractical." *Library Journal* 97 (October 15, 1972):1422.

3. Cheshier, Robert G. "Fees for Services in Medical Library Networks." *Bulletin of the Medical Library Association* 60 (April 1972):325–32.

4. "NLM to Charge Fees for MEDLINE Service." *Library Journal* 98 (May 1, 1973):1422.

5. Berry, John N. "Double Taxation." *Library Journal* 101 (November 15, 1976):2321.

6. Blake, Fay M., and Perlmutter, Edith L. "The Rush to User Fees: Alternative Proposals." *Library Journal* 102 (October 1, 1977):2005–8.

7. Surprenant, T.T. "Future Libraries." *Wilson Library Bulletin* 58 (April 1984):547–5.

8. Crawford, Paula J., and Thompson, Judith A. "Free Online Searches are Feasible." *Library Journal* 104 (April 1, 1979):793–5.

9. Linford, John. "To Charge or Not to Charge: A Rationale." *Library Journal* 102 (October 1, 1977):2009–10.

10. Killebrew, Marilyn Gill. "User Fees I: The Economic Agreement." *Library Journal* 104 (January 1, 1979):19–22; "User Fees II: The Library Response." *Library Journal* 104 (January 15, 1979):170–3.

11. King, Donald W. "Pricing Policies in Academic Libraries." *Library Trends* 28 (Summer 1979):47–62.

12. Drake, Miriam. "User Fees: Aid or Obstacle to Access." *Wilson Library Bulletin* 58 (May 1984):632–5.

13. Spencer, Carol C. "Unit Costs of Interlibrary Loans and Photocopiers at a Regional Medical Library: Preliminary Report." *Bulletin of the Medical Library Association* 58 (April 1970):189–90.

14. Association of Research Libraries. *A Study of the Characteristics, Costs and Magnitude of Interlibrary Loans in Academic Libraries.* Westport, Connecticut: Greenwood Press, 1972.

15. "Fees for Interlibrary Loans Spread: Scholars Fear Work Will Suffer." *Chronicle of Higher Education* (October 19, 1979) :1.

16. Schultz, Claire K. "Establishing Cost Centers Within Libraries of Medical Centers." *Bulletin of the Medical Library Association* 71 (January 1983) :1–5.

17. Lyders, Richard A. et al. "Cost Allocation and Cost Generation." In: American Library Association. Association of College and Research Libraries. *New Horizons for Academic Libraries,* ed. by R.D. Stueart and R.J. Johnson. Saur Verlag, 1979, 116–22.

18. Kantor, Paul B. "Cost and Usage of Health Sciences Libraries: Economic Aspects." *Bulletin of the Medical Library Association* 72 (July 1984):274–86.

19. Spencer, Carol C. "Random Time Sampling with Self-Evaluation for Library Cost Studies: Unit Costs of Reference Questions." *Bulletin of the Medical Library Association* 68 (January 1980):53–7.

20. Cable, Leslie G. "Cost Analysis to Outside Users." *Bulletin of the Medical Library Association* 68 (April 1980):247–8.

The MEDLARS Pricing Algorithm

Carolyn B. Tilley
David Kenton

ABSTRACT. This paper discusses the rationale used by the National Library of Medicine (NLM) in changing its online pricing scheme, or algorithm, from connect hour only to a component pricing algorithm. It also discusses the implementation of this new pricing method. Before discussion of the new online pricing scheme, a brief history of the NLM online services and charging is included. NLM feels that the algorithm allows for a more equitable way of charging for its online services and also allows for better system usage measurement.

GENERAL HISTORY

The National Library of Medicine (NLM) began experimenting with online bibliographic search services in the fall of 1967. Before that, in 1964, NLM began to use a computerized system for the production of *Index Medicus* and for individualized "demand" searches of the *Index Medicus* database.

Carolyn B. Tilley is Head of the MEDLARS Management Section (MMS) at the National Library of Medicine, 8600 Rockville Pike, Bethesda, MD 20209. Ms. Tilley received her B.S. from American University and her M.L.S. from the University of Maryland. The MEDLARS Management Section, part of the Bibliographic Services Division, serves as the public contact point for the day-to-day operation of the NLM Online User Network. The Section provides answers to telephone and written inquiries about the use and characteristics of the various NLM databases, maintains billing records, processes applications for access to the Network, handles the mailing of offline prints and offsearches, produces manuals and other descriptive materials, and is responsible for all training in the use of the online system.

David Kenton is a Senior Systems Analyst at the National Library of Medicine with primary responsibility for the software management of MEDLINE and technical liaison with the external agencies, both foreign and domestic, which receive MEDLARS databases and software. Mr. Kenton was a member of the design team which developed the original ELHILL/ORBIT software for the System Development Corporation in the early 1970s. He holds a B.A. in Mathematics from the University of Connecticut and originally worked in Air Defense, Intelligence, and Command/Control Systems.

After receipt in the mail of literature search requests, these searches were processed in batches against the entire file. The computer system, called the Medical Literature Analysis and Retrieval System (MEDLARS), began to expand with the growth of the biomedical literature and with the increasing number of demand searches processed. The term MEDLARS still refers to the entire NLM system of over twenty bibliographic citation and non-bibliographic databases. Obtaining a demand search, from request to formulation, to computer processing and mailing, was slow and expensive, taking up to several weeks. In January 1970, NLM began publication of *Abridged Index Medicus* (*AIM*), which is an index to articles in approximately one-hundred English-language journals in clinical medicine. The acceptance *AIM* received from the biomedical community encouraged NLM to choose this small database for an initial pilot study of online services. Arrangements were made to connect a computer at the System Development Corporation (SDC) in California to the Teletypewriter Exchange Network (TWX). The AIM-TWX service, which became operational in June 1970 at about ninety medical institutions, was received with enthusiasm and demonstrated the viability of an online nationwide network. However, AIM-TWX participants expressed a need for a larger database and a less costly method of access.

After a sixteen-month experiment with the AIM-TWX prototype system, MEDLINE (*MEDLARS onLINE*) was made available to the biomedical community in October 1971. It was the first nationally available, local-call, online retrieval system. The initial user group of twenty-five institutions had grown to ninety-two by the end of the first year; by May 1984, there were over 2,300 U.S. users. Non-U.S. MEDLARS centers include Australia, the Pan American Health Organization, Canada, Colombia, France, Kuwait, West Germany, Italy, Japan, Mexico, South Africa, Sweden, Switzerland, and the United Kingdom.

In addition to MEDLINE, more than twenty other databases have been added to MEDLARS during these last ten years. These databases include files providing coverage back through 1966 as well as specialized files in chemistry, toxicology, bioethics, cancer, history of medicine, population, biomedical audiovisuals, and health planning and administration. The NLM catalog, name authority file, Medical Subject Headings (MeSH) vocabulary file, and serials collection are also available to online users.

CHARGING HISTORY

Charging for NLM online services began in August 1973. The initial charge for each aggregate hour a searcher was connected to the system (connect hour) was $6.00. Each page printed offline was charged at ten cents. In 1974, the connect hour charge rose to $15 per hour and in 1975, prime and non-prime hours were introduced to more evenly distribute the searching load on the computer system. Prime-time was defined as 10:00 a.m. ET-5:00 p.m. ET. In 1978, a "lunchtime" period of non-prime time was introduced to try to promote and spread the load of searching during this non-peak system period each day. The hours for this non-prime period were 11:30 a.m.-1:00 p.m. ET. This midday non-prime time was eliminated in 1980 because of low interest. The connect hour charges continued to change in order to recover system costs to the government. Royalties for some databases were introduced and increased somewhat over the years. Royalties are paid to various producers for subfiles included in some NLM databases. The simple flat rate of charging for online hourly usage continued through the 1970s and early 1980s until NLM determined that the connect hours as a measure of usage was no longer valid, both in terms of reporting system usage/growth and as an equitable means of charging for online services.

RATIONALE FOR CHANGE

NLM accumulated connect hours for use as growth indicators and billing by gathering all the minutes spent online by users searching the MEDLARS databases. These connect hours taken over time were used to measure system use. During the 1970s, measuring by connect hour was the best indicator of system usage and growth. However, because of changes in the NLM computer systems and terminal operating speeds, use of only connect hours to measure online services led to an under-representation of actual system growth and service provided.

The growth of technology is mainly responsible for changing the value of the connect hour as a good measure of system usage. In 1971, NLM began operation of ELHILL II with an IBM 370/155 Uniprocessor computer. During the 1970s, NLM's program software became more efficient, the number and types of services increased, databases were added, and system hardware was constantly upgraded. In 1975, MEDLARS II was implemented with a new retrieval system, ELHILL III, on an IBM 370/158 Multiprocessor computer (two central processor units hooked together). During the period 1975–1980, the ELHILL software was further enhanced, more databases were added, disks with greater storage capacities and speeds were added, and better computer hardware was acquired. Also, multiple copies of the ELHILL software program were introduced to speed response time for searchers. In March 1980, ELHILL 3.2 was implemented and in December 1980 an IBM 370/168 computer system was installed.

This software gave NLM system searchers the ability to save and execute entire search formulations online in multiple files. The SAVESEARCH macro capability greatly changed user interaction dynamics, thus dramatically changing the makeup of work accomplished during a connect hour. Instead of keying a search strategy formulation repetitively in each file, searchers now could build a search strategy once, save it, and then execute it successively in various other files by simply entering one SAVESEARCH name during each file connection. By August 1982, NLM had replaced the 370/168 Multiprocessor machine with an IBM 3033 Multiprocessor which is still in use. The 370/168 computer had tripled the processing power available while the 3033 system doubled that processing power.

Other events affected the connect hour: terminal speeds and microcomputer technology. Terminal operating speeds increased from ten to fifteen characters per second (cps), first to 300 baud (30 cps) in the 1970s and then to 1200 baud (120 cps—four times faster) in the early 1980s. These faster speeds allowed some MEDLARS searchers to accomplish more in fewer connect hours. Costs to access the system were no longer being equitably distributed among the users. Searchers with higher speed terminals were accomplishing more and paying proportionately less. Also, the increasing use of programmable microcomputers allowed for even more work to be accomplished in a connect hour. This is because search strategies can be pre-sorted for interrogating the databases and microcomputer software used to quickly download large volumes of data onto disks for later processing and formatting.

The NLM has always carefully monitored the use of its computer system and databases. When the connect hour began to cease being an accurate measure of online service provided, NLM began study to find new and better ways to measure online activity and equitably distribute service costs to searchers.[1]

IMPLEMENTATION

In a letter sent in June 1983 to NLM domestic searchers notifying them of Registry of Toxic Effects of Chemical Substances and Toxicology Data Bank database price changes, NLM included a brief note about the forthcoming change in the online MEDLARS system pricing.[2] Also, at the 1983 NLM Online Users Meeting, held as an unofficial meeting each year at the annual meeting of the Medical Library Association, NLM staff discussed the new pricing algorithm in terms of its three components. These components are connect hour use (which was reduced from previous connect hour charges), work performed by the computer, and characters sent to the user's terminal. Other charges, such as offline processing, page charges, and the monthly minimums for each access code, were not changed.

During the winter of 1983, the programming work for the new algorithm was accomplished. During the summer of 1983, NLM staff tested the new pricing algorithm prior to fall implementation. Based upon usage data analyzed, NLM found that most of its users would experience no increase in overall charges for service. However, those searchers who made extensive use of the system to retrieve and process large numbers of citations (e.g., downloading of citations) would see some increase in their bills. Charges were not increased or decreased per se; rather, the access costs were redistributed among the online users based on actual use of the system and databases rather than on time only. NLM was also careful that the online revenues generated by the new algorithm did not increase, but continued only to recover the costs associated with database access.

The components of the pricing algorithm are:[3]

CONNECT TIME: The algorithm includes an amount for prime and non-prime time connect hours to cover telecommunications costs. Royalty or use charges, when applicable, are included in this component.

COMPUTER WORK: Users are charged for the actual computer work, i.e., entering a search statement, carriage return (interactions), citations printed, and disk accesses (accesses to a disk for the retrieval of citations, commonly referred to as input/output operations). Computer work is only one component of the total charge and generally does not influence a user's bill by more than ten percent to fifteen percent at any given time.

CHARACTERS
PRINTED: A charge is made for the number of characters prepared for transmission to the user's terminal. PRINT commands have the greatest effect on the amount of this charge. Users printing a large number of citations or downloading pay proportionately. Two users, one using a 300 baud terminal and the other a 1200 baud terminal, will pay the same amount for characters transmitted to the terminal regardless of the speed of transmission.

To reduce costs for searchers when using ELHILL information commands (to view non-bibliographic material), NLM introduced a file called INFORM. This file allows users to issue EXPLAIN commands and to read the online NEWS items without incurring character charges. EXPLAINing a database or a system feature or viewing the online NEWS involves transmission of a large number of characters. NLM did not feel it fair to charge by characters for these types of activities.

THE SHOW COST COMMAND

To familiarize searchers with the cost components of the new algorithm and to provide them with a way of estimating costs for online searches, NLM introduced the SHOW COST command on its computer. In the July 1983 *NLM Technical Bulletin,* an article explained the command and its use.[4] Prior to the implementation of the component algorithm in the fall, the SHOW COST command facilitated the display of costs based on the connect hour charges only which were then in effect for online MEDLARS services. There are two types of SHOW COST commands: those related to a database and those related to an entire terminal session. The database commands display cumulated totals and costs for searching a database; that is, from time of initial login into a particular database until the issuance of a FILE command (to change files) or a logoff command (STOP Y). Session commands display cumulative totals and costs for all databases from initial login until a STOP Y logoff command is input.

```
The SHOW COST commands are:

SHOW COST
                              DATABASE COMMANDS
SHOW COST DETAILED


SHOW COST TOTAL
                              SESSION COMMANDS
SHOW COST TOTAL DETAILED
```

DATABASE COMMANDS:

```
USER:
SHOW COST
PROG:
THE ESTIMATED TOTAL ONLINE COST FOR THIS 16 MINUTE MEDLINE SESSION IS $5.87.
```

```
USER:
SHOW COST DETAILED
PROG:
THE ESTIMATED TOTAL ONLINE COST FOR THIS 16 MINUTE MEDLINE SESSION IS $5.87.
YOU HAVE ENTERED 8 INTERACTIONS AND 5 SEARCH STATEMENTS.
3 CITATIONS WERE PRINTED AND 1638 CHARACTERS WERE SENT TO YOUR TERMINAL.
THE COMPUTER HAS USED 690 WORK UNITS IN PERFORMING YOUR INTERACTIONS.
```

SESSION COMMANDS:

```
USER:
SHOW COST TOTAL
PROG:
THE ESTIMATED TOTAL ONLINE COST FOR THIS 18 MINUTE TERMINAL SESSION IS $6.75.
```

```
USER:
SHOW COST TOTAL DETAILED
PROG:
THE ESTIMATED TOTAL ONLINE COST FOR THIS 16 MINUTE TERMINAL SESSION IS $5.91.
YOU HAVE ENTERED 10 INTERACTIONS AND 3 SEARCH STATEMENTS.
15 CITATIONS WERE PRINTED AND 1240 CHARACTERS WERE TRANSMITTED TO YOUR TERMINAL.
THE COMPUTER HAS USED 651 WORK UNITS IN PERFORMING YOUR TRANSACTIONS.
```

Various options for SHOW COST include abbreviations, optional punctuation (commas), and a RESET facility to allow the database "counters" to be reset to zero. The RESET feature is especially useful when a searcher is performing multiple searches for different requesters in one database. By using RESET after each search, discrete cost estimates for each patron's search in that particular database may be provided. RESET can also be used with session commands but will reset counters for only the database currently in use by the searcher.

When a logoff command, STOP Y, is issued, the program automatically generates a SHOW COST TOTAL display. In addition, the message '***END OF SESSION***' is displayed after the GOOD-BYE message and a final, total session cost display is issued by the system. All cost information shown by the command are estimates only. Charges included in the actual invoices may differ slightly from the online estimates. Charges associated with OFFSEARCHes and other offline processes are not included in SHOW COST displays but are part of the monthly invoice or statements of account.

The component charging went into effect in October 1983 (April 1984 for non-U.S. partners). Table 1 shows the current algorithm prices for online services.

COST-EFFECTIVE SEARCHING

NLM continues to monitor system and database usage. Several articles with guidelines for cost-effective searching have been published, and will continue to be published, in the *NLM Technical Bulletin*.[5,6]

Some tips for cost-effective searching under the new pricing algorithm which were included in the *Bulletin* are summarized below:

1. MEDLARS searchers are encouraged to take advantage of the SAVE and SAVESEARCH capabilities. In general, searches should be formulated in the current or "front" files (i.e., MEDLINE and TOXLINE as opposed to their back-files). After saving search strategies, they should be executed online in the appropriate backfiles. The use of the SAVE-SEARCH macro capability helps to reduce connect and computer work unit charges by minimizing the necessity of re-keying search formulations in each file.

2. To reduce character charges:

• Print only titles and/or vocabulary terms, instead of complete citations thereby reducing character charges, when ascertaining the relevance of retrieval. If titles or MeSH headings confirm that the search needs no further refinement or broadening, the citations may then be printed in the full format desired.
• Use the offline print capability when citations are not needed immediately. Offline printing is generally more cost effective than online printing, but only if the citations are not needed immediately.
• Assess the value of setting the MEDLARS user profile

TABLE 1

NLM ONLINE PRICING ALGORITHM

	CONNECT CHARGE (Per Hour)		SEARCH STATEMENT CHARGE	CITATION CHARGE	INTERACTION CHARGE (Carriage Returns)	COMPUTER RESOURCES (Disk Accesses) (Per 100)		CHARACTER CHARGES (Per 1,000)	
	Non-Prime	Prime				Non-Prime	Prime	Non-Prime	Prime
MEDLINE & BACKFILES	$ 4.50	$ 7.25	$ .01	$ .01	$ .01	$ .06	$ .12	$ .08	$ .12
TOXLINE & BACKFILES	33.87*	36.62*	.01	.07*	.01	.06	.12	.08	.12
CHEMLINE	39.50*	42.25*	.01	.07*	.01	.06	.12	.08	.12
RTECS	39.00	42.75	.01	.01	.01	.06	.12	.08	.12
TDB	56.50	60.25	.01	.01	.01	.06	.12	.08	.12
ALL OTHER	4.50	7.25	.01	.01	.01	.06	.12	.08	.12
MEDLEARN	15.00	22.00	-	-	-	-	-	-	-

*Includes Royalty Charges of $29.37 Per Connect Charge and $0.06 Per Citation for TOXLINE and its Backfiles and $35.00 Per Connect Charge and $0.06 Per Citation for CHEMLINE.

FEDERAL, STATE, AND/OR LOCAL TAXES ARE NOT INCLUDED. TERMINALS AND TELEPHONE/LINE CHARGES ARE THE RESPONSIBILITY OF THE CENTER. CURRENT PRIME TIME IS 10:00 A.M. TO 5:00 P.M. MONDAY THROUGH FRIDAY EASTERN TIME. ALL OTHER TIME IS NON-PRIME TIME.

area to a shorter page length (the number of lines that print out between the 'CONTINUE PRINTING? (YES/ NO)' messages). The algorithm charges for characters created, or prepared for transmission, to the user's terminal. These characters are prepared in "batches" depending on the PAGELENGTH set in the user profile area. If printing is interrupted by the transmission of the BREAK key, those characters prepared, but not received at the terminal, will be included in the charge for characters. In other words, if a PRINT command is issued and then the BREAK key is depressed before the PRINT is complete, billing will occur for the characters that would have been received at the terminal until a CONTINUE PRINTING? cue appeared, had the BREAK key not been hit. Depending on the style of searching, some users may wish to consider shortening the number of lines (therefore the number of characters) prepared for each PRINT batch. The PAGELENGTH is currently variable, from ten to one hundred lines.

3. To reduce computer work units:

- Use Pre-Explosions (included in the printed *MeSH* thesaurus) when they exist rather than exploding MeSH headings, thus reducing disk accesses.
- Avoid redundant use of explosions or highly posted terms. It is cost-effective to enter an exploded term or a highly posted term in a separate search statement that can be referred to subsequently in combination with other terms.
- Follow stringsearch (character string searching) guidelines whenever possible. Limit retrieval as much as possible, especially with Text Words, before stringsearching. Stringsearch for items that can be searched directly (such as HUMAN or ENG (LA)) only with a retrieval set of fewer than 300 citations. Conversely, search directly for these items with a retrieval set of 300 or more citations. Stringsearch multiple items in a single stringsearch instruction if appropriate.

CONCLUSION

NLM staff believe that the new pricing algorithm for MED-LARS online services is superior to the old connect hour only algorithm. This is true both in terms of charging searchers more equitably for services and in gathering system growth data. NLM also believes that the new pricing algorithm is more "user-friendly." User-friendly, in this case, means that it is now less expensive for a MEDLARS search analyst to sit and think for a few moments while connected online to the system before proceeding with a particular search action. Before the component algorithm was introduced, it was more costly for the terminal operators to sit and collect their thoughts or briefly evaluate further actions while they were connected online to a database. It would have cost, under the old connect hour only algorithm, for MEDLINE during non-prime time, $15 an hour to "think." However, it is now only $4.50 per hour (or seven and one-half cents per non-prime MEDLINE minute) for a searcher to pause briefly before proceeding. Also, since factors other than simple time are collected and charged, it is sometimes worthwhile to evaluate certain search actions, such as stringsearching or "exploding" before proceeding.

REFERENCES

1. Kenton, David. "The Development of a More Equitable Method of Billing for Online Services." *ONLINE* 8 (September 1984): 13–7.

2. Colaianni, Lois Ann, and Kissman, Henry. Letter of June 27, 1983, to NLM online searchers. *NLM Technical Bulletin* 170 (June 1983): Enclosure.

3. Colaianni, Lois Ann, and Kenton, David. "New Pricing Algorithm." *NLM Technical Bulletin* 171 (July 1983): 5–6.

4. Colaianni, Lois Ann, and Kenton, David. "The SHOW COST Command." *NLM Technical Bulletin* 171 (July 1983): 7–8.

5. Tilley, Carolyn B., and Proudman, Sheila T. "General Guidelines for Cost-Effective Searching." *NLM Technical Bulletin* 172 (August 1983): 7–9.

6. Tilley, Carolyn B. "Search Hint: Tips for Cost-Effective Searching under the New Pricing Algorithm." *NLM Technical Bulletin* 173 (September 1983): 7–9.

Online Search Services:
A Strategy for Cost Recovery

Marlene Caldwell
Caroline Mann
Bonnie M. Barnard

ABSTRACT. The Houston Academy of Medicine–Texas Medical Center Library recently converted from a fixed-price charging mechanism to a mechanism of direct costs plus a base fee for online searches. Under the new system, all overhead costs are added up and divided by the number of searches. This average figure becomes the base fee which is charged for every unique database search. In addition to the base fee, clients pay only the cost of their individual search, resulting in a more equitable system. Using this system, the effects of vendor price changes are simplified, searchers are allowed their choice of vendor and a variety of client requests can be easily accommodated.

Online search services have become increasingly important in academic health sciences libraries since MEDLINE was first introduced nearly fifteen years ago. Initially, most libraries subsidized the costs of their online search services with institutional funds but because of the increasing demand for

Marlene Caldwell and Caroline Mann coordinate the Automated Information Services at the Houston Academy of Medicine–Texas Medical Center Library.

Marlene Caldwell is an Information Services Librarian at the Houston Academy of Medicine–Texas Medical Center Library. She received her M.L.I.S. from the University of Texas at Austin.

Caroline Mann is an Information Services Librarian at the Houston Academy of Medicine–Texas Medical Center Library. She received her M.S.L.S. from the University of North Carolina at Chapel Hill.

Bonnie M. Barnard is currently the Infection Control/Inservice Education Coordinator at Beltway Community Hospital in Pasadena, Texas. Formerly, she was the Administrative Assistant in the Information Services Department at the Houston Academy of Medicine–Texas Medical Center Library. She received the Master of Public Health degree from the University of Texas Health Science Center at Houston, School of Public Health.

95

online services and the rising costs of databases, equipment, telecommunications, etc., many libraries have had to develop mechanisms for cost recovery.

The Houston Academy of Medicine–Texas Medical Center (HAM-TMC) Library has used various methods of cost recovery for online search services since 1973. Recently, the Library's cost recovery system was reevaluated and after much deliberation, it was switched from a fixed-price structure to a base fee plus direct cost structure. This paper will focus on the rationale that led to that change, the actual steps taken to implement the change and the reactions of both library staff and clients.

The HAM-TMC Library is unusual among medical libraries in the United States in that it is a consortium library. Not affiliated directly with a single educational institution, it receives support from nineteen institutions whose faculty, students, and staff depend on the Library for health sciences-related information. Each institution is assessed an annual fee to suport the Library and its services. The Library's clientele (15,000 registered cardholders) is represented by individuals from two medical schools, three nursing schools, several hospitals, other health-related agencies, the local medical society, law firms, and the general public.

Cardholders at the HAM-TMC Library are eligible to use the Library and all of its services; however, there are fees for services tailored to a client's specific needs, such as photocopying and formal computer searches. The Library receives approximately 350 formal computer search requests per month. In addition, Information Services Librarians use the computer to assist with approximately one hundred reference questions each month and also to run about seventy-five short (quick and dirty) searches. Cardholders receive reference and short searches free of charge.

IDENTIFICATION OF THE PROBLEM

MEDLINE searches using the National Library of Medicine (NLM) system have traditionally accounted for 85 percent to 90 percent of all searches done at the HAM-TMC Library. A fixed-price method of charging based on the NLM file structure was developed for these searches several years ago. The charge for a MEDLINE search depended on the inclusion or exclusion of abstracts and the number of years searched. The price breakdown was as follows during the summer of 1983:

	Without Abstracts	With Abstracts
1980-present	$13.00	$16.00
1977-present	18.00	23.00
1975-present	23.00	29.00
1971-present	27.00	34.00
1966-present	33.00	40.00

The fixed-price structure for MEDLINE searches was determined through a rather complex formula based on several averages. The information for these averages was taken from the HAM-TMC Library daily computer search logs, the Automated Information Services (AIS) expense records and database use statistical reports. The averages calculated were: (1) the cost of the average online time for a single search request on the NLM MEDLINE file, (2) the costs of the average number of pages for a current file search using both the standard format and the abstracted format, and (3) the average cost per search for the Library's overhead (telephone, service contracts, supplies, documentation, training, demos, reruns and reference use of the computer). The sum of these averages became the current file charges for a search—$13.00 for the standard format and $16.00 for the abstracted format. Average page costs for each backfile for both types of formats were calculated also and added to the current file costs to determine the charges for backfile searches. All personnel time for searching or administering the service was excluded from the formula because the Library recovers personnel costs through the basic institutional assessments.

The fixed-price system applied to all MEDLINE searches, irrespective of the vendor used. For all other NLM databases a per minute fee was computed based on the connect hour costs and the Library's overhead costs. For non-NLM files the average overhead costs became a base fee which was added to the direct costs (vendor/producer charges) for the search.

In effect, there were three separate charge structures for computer searches at the HAM-TMC Library in the summer of 1983—one for MEDLINE searches, one for the other NLM databases, and one for non-NLM databases. Oddly enough, the triple structure was simple to use in many ways because only 10 percent to 15 percent of the searches fell outside the fixed-price system. Under the fixed-price system, clients knew the cost of their search before the search was run. As many as 300 citations per file could be printed for the quoted price; when the number of citations exceeded 300 there was only a slight increase in price. Also, the online time pressure for the Library's search analysts was minimal since the price of the search was not dependent on the actual execution time.

However, there were some very obvious problems with this triple price structure and particularly with the fixed-priced system. Each time NLM increased its prices or reconfigured its files, there was a time consuming recalculation of the Library's price structure. When NLM announced its intention to switch to the current pricing algorithm, Library staff felt that the fixed-price system was too complex to accommodate this change. Also, searchers at the HAM-TMC Library were becoming less and less dependent on NLM for MEDLINE searches, and more frequently searching on other vendor systems. Conforming to a price structure based on the NLM MEDLINE file configuration when searching other systems made the fixed-price system cumbersome and artificial. The fixed-price system also required clients to tailor their search requests to NLM's year configuration. For example, if a client wanted a search from 1976 to the present, they would pay the 1975 to present rate for that search. Another problem was the occasional request for one of the backfiles without the current file, because all of the overhead was calculated into the current file. Because the fixed-price system was based on the assumption of a fifteen-minute online search, searchers were reluctant to do much online printing. Unless there was an urgent need for the material, the search was printed offline. In short, under the fixed-price system requesters had to fit into the Library's specifications instead of the Library trying to tailor the search to users' needs.

Finally, the strongest objection to the fixed-price system

was that clients were paying for the average search, not for what their search actually cost. Searchers felt the system was not as equitable as it should be. Clients requesting a search on a narrow subject with few hits were in fact helping to finance broad comprehensive searches. This system was particularly hard on students, a population the Library encourages to use the search service.

STRATEGY FOR THE DEVELOPMENT OF A NEW SYSTEM

It was clear that the Library needed to explore alternative pricing structures for the search service. Given the problems previously mentioned, searchers established the following criteria for a new pricing structure:

1. Cost equality: clients should pay only the cost incurred by their requests
2. Ease of use for Library staff and clientele

   a. Internal use of one bookkeeping system for all searches irregardless of vendor or database
   b. Simple internal accounting procedures for billing computer searches

3. Sensitivity to vendor price changes
4. Freedom to choose any vendor
5. Flexibility to accommodate various types of search requests
6. Cost recovery of the Library's overhead

Before proceeding, AIS staff consulted other libraries and found quite a variety of fee structure in use. The structures fell into two categories: those similar to the fixed-price structure and those that used formulas broken down to a "per minute" charge. It also was discovered that some search services were still partially subsidized and thus able to offer searches at very attractive low prices. None of these alternative fee structures seemed to meet enough of the Library's basic criteria and because only personnel costs are subsidized through the institutional assessment, the Library's search service must recover all other costs associated with it.

THE NEW SYSTEM

After reevaluating the present triple-structured system, it became apparent that the Library's method of charging for non-NLM searches fit the desired criteria for the new system. It was simple, equitable and flexible. Overhead costs were averaged into a base fee that was the same for every search. All direct costs of the search (online time, royalties, and page or citation charges) were charged to individual clients. This became the model for the Library's new system.

The new system required an accountability for total overhead costs. The HAM-TMC Library is fortunate to have an accountant who issues monthly reports of all AIS expenses separate from the rest of the Library budget. From these reports exact figures on communications, education and training, equipment, printing, service contracts, supplies and miscellaneous expenses were obtained. Another overhead expense was the cost of reruns, demonstrations, reference searches and short searches. These two groups of overhead expenses from the previous year were added together and that figure was divided by the number of paid searches for that year. The base fee is the average cost per search for overhead expenses associated with the search service.

$$\frac{\text{overhead expenses for one year}}{\text{\# of paid searches for one year}} = \text{base fee per search}$$

Following the above formula, the Library determined the base fee to be $7.00 per search. This was not a significant change from what had been charged as the base fee for the non-NLM database searches under the triple-structured system. Under this new system, clients now bear equal financial responsibility for maintaining the search service (base fee) and pay for the actual information they require (direct costs of the search).

IMPACT OF THE NEW SYSTEM

Introducing a price change is never easy since it affects the Library's clients and staff. One difficult aspect of the new system is that it is no longer possible to tell clients the exact cost of their search when taking the request. Now, searchers spend more time during the interview discussing the various price components of a search and answering general questions about the search service. (A handout was designed to assist with this and it is available at the Information Services desk.) Initial fears that an "up front" base fee would deter clients never materialized. Reaction to the change has been minimal—computer request statistics have remained constant and searchers have detected no negative feedback about the base fee. This is probably because there was not an actual price increase, but just a change in the pricing mechanism. Also, many of the Library's clients are becoming more knowledgeable about the costs associated with computers and searching.

The major advantage of the new system is that searchers can easily accommodate a variety of client requests. Under the old system searchers attempted to confine online printing to emergency cases. With the new system if the client wants citations printed online in spite of the price difference, then searchers are able to provide that service.

The new system allowed AIS to devise an entirely new departmental procedure for administering the search service. The two logbooks were combined into one which simplified logging searches, checking search status, and compiling monthly AIS statistics. New search request forms were designed and printed. Although these forms are more complicated than previous forms, they are "generic" and can accommodate searches on any database or vendor. The front of the form contains the basic request information; the reverse side of the form is a grid for recording data necessary to determine the cost of a search—file name, vendor, online time, online cost, NLM offsearch charges, number of pages, NLM page costs, BRS packet charge and other offline print/citation charges (see Figure 1). Only the categories that apply to the vendor used to search are filled in (e.g., the NLM categories are left blank when a search is run on BRS). The base fee or

#	Database	System Vendor	Online Time	Online Cost	NLM off chg	(NLM) #pp	(NLM) $pp	BRS 50c pkg	Other off chg	Service Charge	Sub Total Cost	Non Card $20	Non-Chg Cost	GRAND TOTAL
				$	$	$	$	$	$	$	$	$	$	$
1										$7.00			-	
2										$7.00			-	
3										$7.00			-	
4										$7.00			-	
5										$7.00			-	
6										$7.00			-	
7										$7.00			-	
8										$7.00			-	
9										$7.00			-	
10										$7.00			-	

FIGURE 1

service charge is printed on the form as a reminder to searchers to add it to the cost for each database search. The search form also contains a category for not charging a portion of the overall cost of the search if the situation warrants it. The noncharge amount, if any, is left to the discretion of the searcher. Including this option has been especially useful when training new searchers. It also has reduced the searchers' fears of incurring excessive online costs when faced with situations such as slow response time or being dropped by the system. Having worked under a fixed-price system where the "average search" was presumed to take about fifteen minutes, some searchers were not aware of their individual average search time. The fears that some searchers had about spending too much time online or being under too much pressure haven't been realized so far. On the contrary it seems as though the new system has been a confirmation of their efficiency in performing searches. When it has been necessary, however, a portion of the costs have been charged back to the Library on the request form. However, the amount per person has been negligible so far.

The record keeping, though combined into one system for all databases, is much more complex. In order to monitor ongoing expenses and income in a timely manner, it is necessary to record more data about each search. At the end of each month the administrative secretary collects all the data and creates an expense report. The support staff is responsible also for keeping all log books, sorting the printoffs and adding up the cost of each search.

The new system has had a few minor surprises. No one in Information Services realized that varying prices for computer searches would affect the Circulation staff. On the first day of the new procedure, a client paid for a search at the Circulation Desk with $15.42 in cash. The immediate result was a rather frustrated call from a Circulation staff member. It seemed that only a few pennies were kept in the cash register because they were infrequently needed under the old pricing system. Obviously the new price structure would affect stocking the cash register. To remedy the situation, it was decided to round search charges to the nearest nickel.

CONCLUSION

The method of charging for any of the HAM-TMC Library services undergoes constant review and evaluation. In a year, if it is found that AIS is not recovering the online search service costs, the base fee will be raised to cover those costs. With the advent of in-house versions of MEDLINE the costs of providing computer searches may become less of an issue. For now, however, AIS has settled on a charging mechanism that seems both equitable for clients and financially workable for the Library.

The Entrepreneurial Hospital Library

Jacqueline D. Bastille

ABSTRACT. As our society moves into the information age we are shifting into an age of self-help. The health care industry is changing from a professionally driven industry to a consumer driven one. To respond effectively to the changes which are resulting in decreased budgets and increased demands for information, the hospital library must retool financially to operate as a business. The actual cost of providing access to information as well as services should be analyzed, and allocated or billed to users as a means to gain self-sufficiency. To be successful the entrepreneurial library will have to strive for management excellence and refined marketing skills. This new view of the library combined with the new electronic technology should allow us to serve users with a consistently high level of satisfaction.

INTRODUCTION

As this society moves into the information era, it is shifting from a managerial orientation to an entrepreneurial orientation. As large organizations struggle with the enormous pressures for change brought on by the new technology, only the individual or the small group can be relied on to solve immediate problems. This is an age of self-help when entrepreneurship blooms.[1]

The outside forces that are stimulating change in the society are right now changing the way health care is delivered, how it is marketed, and how it is financed. The health care

Jacqueline D. Bastille is Director of the Health Sciences Libraries, at the Massachusetts General Hospital in Boston, MA. She has written a course syllabus and a chapter on hospital library space planning, and a syllabus on managing the basic health science library for a course she taught at the Fourth International Medical Library Congress, 1980 in Yugoslavia. This paper is based upon a keynote address entitled "Retooling: Opportunities for Change," presented at the Medical Library Association Mid-Atlantic Chapter Meeting, November 3, 1983.

industry is changing from a professionally driven industry to a consumer driven one. Hospitals are analyzing their market shares, identifying what they do best at least cost, even talking about charging actual costs for low-volume procedures rather than subsidizing them by income from high-volume low cost procedures. Patterns of care are shifting from the in-hospital base to the out-patient. Each health care stop, doc in the box, or surgicenter will require fast, easy, and cheap access to information as will hospitals with in-patients in order to guarantee cost-effective patient care.

And so the hospital library must change as its market is changing and expanding. In order to be able to change and to offer information service to this broader marketplace the primary task of the library is to retool financially, that is, to find new creative ways of funding its operations.

THE ENTREPRENEURIAL LIBRARY

The traditional view of the library is that it is an educational agency organized for the general good of society or the institution which it serves, to provide books, journals, and media free of charge to its constituents. Hospital libraries have long tried to serve the needs of many with too little money.

The Medical Library Assistance Act of 1965 tried to remedy this by pumping money into the library system, with the intention of stimulating more sophisticated information service supported by greatly strengthened library budgets. This was very successful for a while. Certainly the number and size of hospital libraries have increased. And they have provided more sophisticated information service supported by greatly strengthened library budgets which grew in the seventies in places where there had previously been none. But now hospital libraries are in trouble again. The growth of the budget has halted but the need, the demand, and the cost of information continues to mushroom. A new way must be found to solve the old problems.

It seems clear that the new perspective of the hospital library should be enlarged to that of a not-for-profit business: a business which assigns a value to the access to its resources, a value to its services, and to the products it provides; a business which markets all these; a business which charges fees sufficient to adequately cover direct costs, and eventually to totally fund all its operations.

This paradigm shift, this new perspective, also will require that librarians retool their attitudes, their values, and their own self-worth. They will have to stop cringing at the idea of the library as a business: like other businesses, libraries have always had inventories of goods which they serviced for people to use. They will have to estimate the value of what they do for their users and carefully explore what their users value versus what the librarians think they should value. And if they are to successfully sell their information services they will have to perceive themselves as well worth the fee they must charge.

Over the last decade, librarians have been urged to use business techniques to run their libraries: to develop appropriate goals by asking themselves what business they are in, to develop skills in marketing their services, and to use budgeting techniques used by profit-making organizations. Now libraries must not only act like businesses but become businesses. Hospitals are businesses. If they had been operating all along as such, there might not be as much panic over the regulatory cost controls as exists in the health care industry today. Hospital administrators are very much aware of this fact. Also businesses are universities, museums, cultural centers, and voluntary associations.

To become a business the library should be totally self-supporting. This may not be possible or even practical for many. But libraries must experiment with this approach and move in this direction in order to be free to flexibly respond to the demands of the user, that is to the library's market. The users will evaluate the worth of the library's services by their willingness to pay for them; they will be voting for them with their money instead of with fine words. Fine words are often discounted by administrators and financial officers when they are asked to approve new programs. Money is never discounted. And so in this information age, the entrepreneurial health sciences library should prosper.

RETOOLING FINANCIALLY

The concept of an entrepreneurial library must be qualified so that it meshes with the present day position of the hospital library in the organization it serves. For many institutions, particularly the small to medium size hospitals, a totally self-supporting library will not be cost-effective, whereas in the large teaching hospitals/medical research centers, the self-supporting library may be highly cost-effective as well as cost-beneficial.

The small organization will find it too costly to bill and account for the sale of services. Nevertheless, the librarian in this type of hospital should analyze all costs for doing business so that the administration will have a clearer picture of actual costs for library services.

First, the costs for marketing resources available for use in the library should be identified. This is called identifying the common load. This can be done easily by doing the following:

1. Conduct a survey of user visits to document number of visits per day, job status and department of users, and reason for visit.
2. Calculate percentage of use by job status, for example residents, or by department, or even by reason for the visit, such as "to get information for a patient care problem."
3. Divide the cost of days open into the annual expense budget minus costs for special services to provide a daily cost of providing access to the library.
4. Divide the cost per day open by the average number of daily visits to calculate the per visit cost.

Next, costs to maintain the "common load" can be displayed according to percentage of use by department, by job status, or by reason for the visit such as patient care, teaching, or research. The data also may be used to determine charges for use of the library by outsiders.

Costs to provide special service such as photocopying, on-line database searches, and citation verfications, should be analyzed to develop a unit cost. This should be done carefully

with the advice of an administrator or a financial person because there are many variables which may be used to develop
costs. For instance, if the user is to be charged for interlibrary
loans should this charge be the amount the library must pay
within the Regional Medical Library Network? Will this fee
cover all the costs incurred such as costs for telephone calls or
online charges to locate a book? If the fee does not cover all
costs should the fee be increased or should the library/hospital
budget subsidize this service? And, finally, is the fee set at a
level which the users can afford, or is it higher than the market will bear?

If users are to be charged for special services it is vital that
convenient and appropriate mechanisms be established for
users to charge or to pay for these. The following scenario
will illustrate the need for these.

A hospital library decided to run a test to see how their
users would react to being charged for quick computer
searches which previously had been free. They started out
charging a cash fee of a nickel per search. Reactions were
immediately loud and angry. And use of the service declined
considerably. After six weeks the cash price was raised to fifty
cents and use fell again to about fifty percent of previous use.

Two large errors were made in the conception of the test.
First, the library required that payment be made in cash.
House Officers, in particular, resented being asked to pay out
of their personal pockets for hospital business, even though
later they were reimbursed by their departments. Second, the
fee of a nickel or even fifty cents was ludicrous to the user for
a product which was worth a great deal more. The very low
fee can imply that the product is really not worth much, or it
can be interpreted as a penalty rather than as a reasonable fee
to cover costs of a worthwhile service. This library now
charges $2 per search, which can be charged back to a depart-
ment cost center. Use of the service has since increased and
according to the librarian is now well respected.

In a large teaching hospital which offers tertiary care and
which is a medical research center, the mix of library users is
complex, as is the source of funds for the institution's budget.
It is usually advantageous for this type of institution to bill and
account for interdepartmental services and to allocate overhead costs to each department. It is equally advantageous for

the library to charge for its services because, for one thing, this provides an evaluation of its services which appears monthly on the library's Expense and Income Statement and which is carefully read by administrators and fiscal officers. In addition, revenue from special research and educational grant funds and from cash payments are usually applied to the library's budget as part of its contribution to the hospital's overhead, thereby reducing the amount the hospital must supply from its operational funds for the library's budgeted expenses. The more income from outside sources the library brings in, the happier is the administration, which classifies the library as a support service which must have all its expenses fully funded by the operational budget of the institution.

PROFILE OF A LARGE LIBRARY

At the Massachusetts General Hospital, the Library is on the hospital's operating budget. Historically about eighty percent of its operating costs have supported information services for patient care and these have been allowed as reimbursable costs by third party health care payers. The remaining twenty percent have been applied to the research overhead costs which are charged to all research grants. In recent years changes have occurred which make this arrangement seem not so beneficial or fair as it had seemed in the past, and which raise questions about how to fairly allocate costs for library services.

A new educational Institute was inaugurated several years ago which grants graduate degrees in nursing and several allied health specialties. This Institute must be clearly self-supporting and its expenses must be kept separate from the hospital's operating budget just as are those of research projects. An estimated fee to cover costs for Library support of the educational programs was agreed upon as the Institute's contribution to the Library's budget. This is treated as revenue from an outside source. Is this amount fair, too much or too little?

Use of the Library for research projects has increased greatly within the last few years as has the cost of the publications required. Should the formula for research overhead costs for the Library be changed? How can this be done fairly and in a way which will benefit all sectors of the hospital whose ultimate focus is on improving the care of the patient?

The third and most restrictive event has been the stringent cost constraints placed on Massachusetts hospital budgets by the state legislature. A regulatory cap was placed on all hospital revenues and expenses using 1981 as a base year. Over a three-year period hospitals must reduce their budgets, both revenues and expenses, by two percent per year. In 1986, it is expected that the hospitals in this state will shift to the Diagnosis Related Group cost basis, which will have a similar budget restricting impact. The effect of the fiscal cap has been to maintain the Library's budget at a status quo level. How can it account for increased use of services which increases both expenses and revenues? How can adequate resources be provided for the growing educational and research programs with a restricted budget governed by patient care fiscal constraints?

Some service units in the hospital such as the Photography Laboratory and the Television Production Unit have been shifted from the operating budget to special funds status which, as for all research projects, requires the Unit to totally support itself. Can the Library as an entrepreneurial agency totally support its operations? The idea is a very attractive one if costs for the common load can be assessed fairly for all sectors of users, and if the Library can successfully sell special services for fees which cover all costs and provide a profit margin.

At present, revenue from outside sources averages about twenty percent of total expenditures. All such income earned by the Library must be applied to its budget expenses as a contribution to the hospital budget as a whole. This means that it cannot use increased income to buy new equipment or additional resources but must, in a sense, donate it to the hospital to help cover the expenses of other units which may not be able to earn income or which may not be able to manage their budgets as effectively.

A subcommittee of the large Library Program Planning Group is exploring the possibilities for changing the allocations of library costs and for shifting the Library from the operating budget to a special fund budget so that profit can be used flexibly to improve service and equipment. It is also reviewing better methods of assessing costs, and ways for the Library to earn money by sharing its expertise and resources. The result of this exercise in creative financing should be a financial plan which will allow an increase in the budget to cover automation costs, which will in turn allow for the development and the sale of sophisticated targeted services for fees based on full cost recovery. The other part of the financial planning task is to look for sources of capital funding. Without such a cushion the so-called entrepreneurial library will fail. It can be called venture or risk capital for starting new services, products or businesses.

TRANSFORMATION

To shift from giving information away to selling information will require a transformation of the user's and of the librarian's concept of library service. In her book *The Aquarian Conspiracy: Personal and Social Transformation in the 1980's,* Marilyn Ferguson outlines the stages of transformation which she describes as a journey without a final destination.

The first stage is an entry point which can be triggered by anything that shakes up the old understanding of the world of old priorities. The entry point may be instituting the first fee for service and receiving positive reactions from users and from the administration.

The second stage is exploration. Some librarians are in this stage now, charging a fee for any number of services, trying to improve the situation rather than transforming it, but finding the library still dependent and restricted as an overhead cost burden.

In the third stage which is integration, the mystery is inhabited, that is the shift or the change is accomplished. In this stage time is spent in the pulling together of loose strands into the new framework, re-evaluating techniques and strategies. This stage will be the test for the success of the entrepreneurial library. Success then leads to the fourth stage which is called conspiracy, in which are discovered sources of power and ways to use power for fulfillment, and in service to others.[2]

It seems reasonable and possible to transform the hospital library into an entrepreneurial library, as an active self-perpetuating agency. As an entry point, the librarian can discuss with administrative and financial officers the potential benefits of developing new ways of funding the library and of building a data base about library service costs and about library users.

Each institution has its own unique features and so financial officers must be creative in handling the institution's money. What may be advantageous for one institution may not be so for another. And similarly, what may be advantageous for the library, may not be so for the hospital. The balance of mutual benefits will determine how far or how fast a library may be able to travel along the way to self-sufficiency. Ferguson stresses the importance of the process: "Goals and end points matter less. Learning is more urgent than storing information. Caring is better than keeping. Means are ends. The journey is the destination."[3]

MANAGEMENT EXCELLENCE AND MARKETING SKILLS

In order to enjoy the process of transformation and to successfully operate the library as a business, the librarian will have to concentrate on developing sophisticated management and marketing skills. A recipe for success is laid out in the book *In Search of Excellence* by Thomas J. Peters and Robert H. Waterman, Jr. This is a report of their study of the most successful United States corporations. The authors identify the following eight characteristics as the basics of management excellence:

1. A bias for action (for getting things done)
2. Close to the customer (with service as the top goal, profitability naturally follows)
3. Autonomy and entrepreneurship (decentralized organization fosters small creative teams)
4. Productivity through people (respecting each individual employee's contribution)
5. Hands on, value driven (explicit attention is paid to the values of the company)

6. Stick to the knitting (stick to what the company knows it can do best)
7. Simple form, lean staff (as the organization grows each area is kept small and simple)
8. Simultaneous loose-tight properties (the company is rigidly controlled and yet at the same time insists on autonomy for and innovation from the rank and file).[4]

Marketing is the key to success of the well managed enterprise. Non-profit organizations have developed active programs to sell their services. Alan Andreasen in an article in the *Harvard Business Review* says that many of these organizations orient their marketing to their product rather than their clients; that is, they first determine how they want to market their organization and its services, and then they turn to analyze their customers to achieve their goals. Good marketing strategy should be oriented toward the clients to boost customer satisfaction and not toward products. The process should begin with the consumer, and marketing techniques should be used which can build support from the users or customers. This strategy will then result in improved cash flow from satisfied users.[5]

CONCLUSION

Change is occurring very fast. The information society is an economic reality. And the emphasis in this new society is shifting from supply (which is what librarians do) to selection (which is what librarians must begin to do more). Naisbitt, in his bestseller *Megatrends,* says that information is an economic entity because it costs something to produce, and because people are willing to pay for it. The value of information is whatever people are willing to pay for it.[6]

The concept of the entrepreneurial library as a self-sufficient, consumer-driven information management center is one that should be implemented by most hospital libraries in a style that most benefits its institution and its community. Quick and easy access to information is vital for the cost-effective delivery of health care and should become an accepted part of that cost.

The librarian who entered this profession out of a strong desire to help should not be put off by the pressure to develop business skills and to commercialize a service which has traditionally been free. IBM makes its profits by emphasizing service and pleasing the client by providing exactly what he needs. The entrepreneurial library should do the same. This transformation will only enhance the old reasons for choosing librarianship as a profession. At last, with an adequate financial base and powerful technology librarians should be able to serve users with greater precision and at a much higher level of user satisfaction than was ever possible when library service was free.

REFERENCES

1. Naisbitt, John. *Megatrends: Ten New Directions Transforming Our Lives.* New York, NY: Warner Books, 1982, pp. 131–57.

2. Ferguson, Marilyn. *The Aquarian Conspiracy: Personal and Social Transformation in the 1980's.* Los Angeles, CA: J.P. Tarcher, Inc., 1980, pp. 89–94.

3. Ibid., p. 101.

4. Peters, Thomas J., and Waterman, Robert H., Jr. *In Search of Excellence: Lessons From America's Best-Run Companies.* New York, NY: Harper and Row, 1982, pp. 13–16.

5. Andreasen, Alan H. "Non-Profits: Check Your Attention to Customers." *Harvard Business Review* 60 (May-June 1982):105–10.

6. Naisbitt. *Megatrends,* p. 36.

Cost Recovery Effort
in a Clinical Librarian Program

ABSTRACT. The University of Connecticut Health Center Library's clinical librarianship program, originally funded by a National Library of Medicine grant, is now operated on a cost recovery basis. The evolution of the service from grant funding to shared funding to cost recovery is described.

BACKGROUND

Clinical librarianship began in the early 1970s with Dr. Gertrude Lamb, Librarian at the Health Sciences Library, University of Missouri, Kansas City, Missouri. Dr. Lamb initiated a program in which medical librarians attended bedside rounds as part of the medical school's teaching program through which clinical instruction was provided to medical students. In this setting, the Clinical Medical Librarian, or clinical librarian (CL), was part of the patient care team. The CL saw patients with the house staff and accepted or determined from context patient care questions that needed further information. The clinical librarian then returned to the library and completed a computer search on MEDLINE to identify relevant journal articles. The CL then evaluated those key articles that directly related to the information needed prior to providing photocopies of the two or three key articles to the house staff. This procedure was to take place within twenty-four hours; clinical librarians were assigned to one hospital service where they had a daily commitment.[1]

Ralph D. Arcari is the Director of the University of Connecticut Health Center Library, Farmington, CT 06032. He received his M.L.S. from Drexel University in Philadelphia.

117

UNIVERSITY OF CONNECTICUT HEALTH CENTER

In 1973, Dr. Lamb became Director of Medical Libraries at Hartford Hospital in Hartford, Connecticut. At that time she and the Director of the Health Center Library, University of Connecticut, Mr. James Morgan, agreed to jointly develop a grant proposal to the National Library of Medicine (NLM) to support clinical librarianship programs at their respective institutions. The proposal was successfully received and the first of two grant funded clinical librarianship programs began in Hartford Hospital and the University of Connecticut's John Dempsey Hospital, Farmington, in 1974.[2] The grant was for two years and followed the model at Kansas City. The first grant placed clinical librarians in Pediatrics, Medicine and Surgery at Hartford Hospital and in Medicine at the John Dempsey Hospital. The focus of the first grant from NLM was to evaluate the influence of a clinical librarian on the patient care information needs of health providers. A second grant was received from the National Library of Medicine for the period 1977 through 1978. The author of this article had succeeded Mr. Morgan at this time. This subsequent grant was designed to evaluate the interdisciplinary nature of information requirements of the hospital patient care team and to assemble a database of questions and relevant clinical journal citations based on the reports of clinical librarians in Medicine, Surgery and Pediatrics at Hartford Hospital, OB/GYN at St. Francis Hospital and Medicine at John Dempsey Hospital. Documentation of the effect of clinical librarianship on patient management at the University of Connecticut Health Center appeared in an article by Scura and Davidoff.[3] An initial evaluation of the cost recovery of the clinical librarian program also has been reported.[4]

REFERENCE SERVICES AND CLINICAL LIBRARIANSHIP AT UCHC

At the conclusion of the second NLM grant, the clinical librarians on grant money were placed on institutional funds at the hospitals in which their programs had been active. At the University of Connecticut Health Center (UCHC) this involved an even division of support for clinical librarianship between the UCHC Library and the UCHC School of Medicine. Costs included salary, fringe benefits, computer searching and photocopying. The Associate Dean in the School of Medicine could justify his School's support for clinical librarianship because of the educational services rendered by the CL to house staff through instruction in the use of clinical literature and preparing MEDLINE search strategies. Clinical librarianship during this period, 1979 through 1981, was limited to Medicine at the John Dempsey Hospital. The structure of the program remained the same. A full-time librarian was on bedside rounds five days a week, seeing patients in the morning with house staff and completing computer searches, literature evaluations and photocopying in the afternoon; the process started over again the following morning. The clinical librarian reported ostensibly to the Reference Department, but operated with relative independence.

In late 1981, the Associate Dean of the School of Medicine at UCHC, notified the UCHC Library Director that the School of Medicine could no longer be relied upon to support a clinical librarianship program. The Library Director was advised to seek funds directly from the department served. At this point, clinical librarianship at UCHC was redesigned. Rather than having a full-time clinical librarian in the hospital's medical service, only a part-time service would be offered with the Library assuming the full costs of personnel and the department served paying for computer searches and photocopying. Moreover, rather than serving only one hospital department, each reference librarian would serve as a part-time clinical librarian. Arrangements were made with Surgery, Pediatrics and Medicine to have a part-time clinical librarian each visiting their hospital floors for rounds once or twice a week. This arrangement proved to be not only financially effective but also structurally more reasonable. The hospital at UCHC is only 235 beds; consequently, there are usually insufficient patient care questions to warrant a full-time clinical librarian. Also, by involving more of the reference librarians, the opportunity for increased exposure to clinical medicine with a concomitant sharing of expertise among the reference staff became available.

By 1983/84 clinical librarianship had evolved at UCHC so

TABLE 1

CLINICAL LIBRARIAN   COMPUTER SEARCHES, 1983/1984

UNIVERSITY OF CONNECTICUT HEALTH CENTER

DEPARTMENT	ANNUAL TOTAL	AVERAGE/MONTH
Medicine	278	23
Pediatrics	249	21
OB/GYN	44	4
Restorative Dentistry	43	4
Nursing	12	1
Total	626	52

that CL services were no longer provided to the Surgery Department, but were provided to OB/GYN, Restorative Dentistry and Nursing. The Surgery Department Head had been at Hartford Hospital previously and preferred no clinical librarian to a part-time clinical librarian. Hartford Hospital, with a significantly larger surgical service, had a full-time clinical librarian. An accommodation could not be reached and OB/GYN replaced Surgery at UCHC. Restorative Dentistry was undertaken by the Reference Department Head and an outreach program to Nursing was developed by the Clinical Librarian also serving Pediatrics. Table 1 indicates the volume of computer searches provided in the UCHC clinical librarian program in 1983/84. The total number indicated, 626, represents 27 percent of the 2,280 computer searches done at the UCHC Library in that year.

COST ANALYSIS

At UCHC for the past three fiscal years, costs for the clinical librarian program as determined by the Library have been limited to computer search costs and photocopying expenses.

Both these costs have been billed to the department receiving clinical librarian services. Photocopy costs have been set at $3.00 per article. This is the same rate as the UCHC photocopy service which includes personnel expenses for pulling the journal, photocopying, reshelving and billing and direct costs for the use of the photocopy equipment as charged by the vendor. Personnel costs for photocopying have been determined by time and volume studies in which each function is correlated with the hourly rate for the individual performing that function (see the Appendix for cost analysis form).

Computer costs for clinical librarian searches have usually been lower than research searches. The latter often involve more variables and terms than searches intended to answer a specific patient care question. At the present time UCHC is only charging departments for the direct computer costs involved in obtaining information in response to questions received in the clinical librarian program. This cost is shown by the vendor, Bibliographic Retrieval Services, after each search done. An additional $10.00 fee is added to all other computer searches done at UCHC to cover terminal depreciation, staff continuing education, computer search manuals and reference materials, maintenance and supplies. The $10.00 fee is waived in order to keep CL costs as low as possible to maintain the Library's presence in departments served where the professional library staff also benefit from the educational exposure to clinical medicine.

DEPARTMENT REACTIONS

Hospital departments at UCHC vary in their ability to support a clinical librarianship program depending on their patient care income. As federal and state regulations on cost containment in health care have become more stringent, funds available for clinical librarianship have decreased. The Library is no longer providing photocopies to any departments but simply responding to patient care questions with computer searches. House staff are expected to get photocopies themselves. Even with the lower rates in place here, Pediatrics has limited their house staff to only seven searches per month and each search must be approved by the Chief

Resident. The benefits to the Library obviously in this case have decreased in direct proportion to the ability of the house staff to request services. Ultimately, as was done with Surgery earlier, Pediatrics may be supplanted by a more responsive department.

CONCLUSION AND FUTURE PERSPECTIVE

The clinical librarian program at UCHC has gone through an evolutionary process. Initially the program was full time and grant funded in one department. Then, although still limited to one department, Medicine, clinical librarianship was supported evenly by both the Library and the School of Medicine. Finally, all reference librarians began to serve as clinical librarians with their salaries paid by the Library and direct costs for computer searches paid by departments.

In retrospect, clinical librarianship successfully united the technology of computer searching and photocopying with patient care information needs. Technology appears to be replacing library computer searching and copying with intelligent work stations in the hospital through which house staff can determine or request library holdings and services. The clinical librarian would seem to be a likely candidate for the librarian as information consultant in the electronically networked environment of the twenty-first century academic health center.

REFERENCES

1. Algermissen, Virginia. "Biomedical Librarians in a Patient Care Setting at the University of Missouri-Kansas City School of Medicine." *Bulletin of the Medical Library Association* 62 (October 1974):354–8.

2. "And now, 'clinical librarans' on rounds." *JAMA* 230 (October 28, 1974):521.

3. Scura, Georgia, and Davidoff, Frank. "Case-Related Use of the Medical Literature; Clinical Librarian Services for Improving Patient Care." *JAMA* 245 (January 2, 1981):50–2.

4. Arcari, Ralph D. "Clinical Librarian Program-Cost Recovery Effort." *Clinical LIbrarian Quarterly* 1 (December 1982):7–10.

APPENDIX

UNIVERSITY OF CONNECTICUT HEALTH CENTER LIBRARY

PHOTOCOPY REQUEST COSTS ANALYSIS

EMPLOYEE	OPERATION	NO. OF REQUESTS	TIME SPENT in minutes	TIME/REQUESTS in minutes
1. Clerk	a. Alphabetize and sorts requests	_____	_____	_____
	b. Pull journal from shelf	_____	_____	_____
	c. Photocopy article	_____	_____	_____
	d. Check for items not on shelf	_____	_____	_____
	e. Preliminary organization of bills	_____	_____	_____
	f. Reshelving	_____	_____	_____
2. Administrative Assistant	Billing	_____	_____	_____

COST CALCULATIONS

1. (clerical salary by minute)* x (total no. of minutes/request)   _____

2. (administrative assistant salary by minute)* x (total no. of minutes/request)   _____

Total Cost Per Request   _____

*includes fringe benefits, sick time and vacation

III. MARKETING REFERENCE SERVICES

Marketing focuses on the user's needs. A total marketing program consists of product, place, promotion and price, commonly referred to as the four P's. Bell presents a comprehensive review of marketing reference services, including both theoretical aspects and practical applications for marketing. Lemkau, Burrows and La Rocco describe the development of a successful marketing program for an information service offered to health professionals outside a medical center. The evolution of a marketing program for a fee-based information service is detailed by Freeman and O'Connell.

Marketing Reference Services: Translating Selected Concepts Into Action for a Specific Practice Setting

Jo Ann Bell

ABSTRACT. The application of marketing concepts to library operations enables librarians to structure library services into an integrated whole focused on user's needs. Promotion alone is not adequate. Library services should be seen as a total market offering, based on the benefits and satisfactions which are desired by consumers and designed to meet specific consumer expectations in regard to quality, the service encounter, distribution, and price. Promotion is used to ensure that consumers are aware of product availability and to create the library's image in the consumer's mind.

INTRODUCTION

"Marketing" often conveys the idea of a slick Madison Avenue "wheeler-dealer" or the equally repugnant gaudy used car salesman who says, "Have I got a DEAL for YOU!" In fact, marketing is much more than advertising hype. Exchange is the central concept of marketing. Commonly used definitions of marketing describe it as ". . .activities that direct the flow of goods and services from producer to consumer,"[1] or as ". . .activities necessary. . .to bring about exchange relationships."[2] Exchange involves giving one thing in return for another. An effective marketing program will be

Jo Ann Bell is Director, Health Sciences Library, East Carolina University, Greenville, NC 28734. She received a B.A. from Duke University, an M.L.S. and Ph.D. from the University of North Carolina at Chapel Hill, and an M.B.A. from East Carolina University. She is the author of 11 professional journal articles, two reviews, and a chapter in a monograph, and has written the MLA CE text on marketing.

127

concerned with identifying and carrying out those activities which will result in the library supplying to its clients products which will meet their needs. In return, the library will receive the clients' support as evidenced by the use of its products, by budget allocations, payment of fees, and general support of the library as a significant component of the institution.

Even those of us who are familiar with the marketing concept have a tendency to take an enthusiastic but overly simplistic view of what is involved in marketing. Although services and products are promoted, appropriate criteria are not always applied to their development, distribution, and pricing. All of these components must be considered in the development of an integrated, differential marketing program.

There are a number of obstacles which must be overcome in the development of a marketing program. Many librarians have a negative attitude about marketing, seeing it only as advertising or as an attempt to transfer a concept from the profit sector to the nonprofit sector. Further, each library department has its own goals; often these are incompatible with each other and may be counterproductive to the aims of the marketing program. Finally, often the marketing program is not coordinated or planned; rather it is implemented in a piecemeal or random fashion.[3]

If a health sciences library is committed to applying marketing to its operations, it is important to realize early on that reference and other public services constitute only one component of the library's total marketing program. Indeed, if public services are seen as the only aspects of library operations concerned with marketing, the library's marketing program will be ineffective.

MARKETING SERVICES

A service is defined as an "activity that has value to a buyer."[4] A good is a physical object. Public service activities of libraries include both physical objects and activities which have value for consumers. For instance, a computer search consists of more than just an activity which has value for a buyer; specifically, it includes the librarian's use of his/her knowledge of databases and expertise in accessing them, as well as the attendant equipment. At the same time, a physical object, the printout, is produced. Therefore, this particular product appears to involve both a service and a good. Brown and Fern have suggested two other definitions which may be useful when evaluating the differences in marketing goods and services. "The core offering is either the activity or the physical object including the attendant services. . . .The total market offering is the aggregate of all of the benefits the customer receives as a result of the core offering plus all the values added by members of the marketing channel."[5] This may seem a bit vague and perhaps irrelevant. But, look at a computer search, including the actual options available from the vendor and the library, such as the bibliographic citations, as well as the abstract, as a core offering. The total market offering includes not only the benefits which are available as part of the core offering, but it encompasses also those which are available because the product has been obtained in a given library and the service performed by a specific librarian. This might include the librarian's attitude, knowledge, and approachability, as well as the physical facility, the library's general image/reputation, and the convenience of acquiring the product. The total market offering concept points out the interrelationships which must be taken into account when a marketing program is designed.

A number of distinctions between marketing services and goods have been emphasized in the marketing literature. Although some of these assumptions are being questioned, it is useful to look at those which apply to marketing library services. [5,6,7,8]

Services are intangible. We can describe the output of the service, but it is difficult to describe the input—what is necessary for the creation of the product. Further, it is difficult to describe the benefits in a way that the consumer or potential consumer will have a concrete idea of what he/she will receive. Reference services, even answering a relatively "simple" question, are representative of the problems encountered. There may be a great deal of data massaging going on in the librarian's brain, even though the response to the question may be almost instantaneous. The consumer does not see this process and in the case of the simpler question is unaware of it, but this is the service. The service is the intellectual process which accesses a data bank in a systematic, yet random manner, and identifies the appropriate source for supplying the desired information.

In addition, the specific benefit for the consumer, whether it be saving time or even improved access to the desired information, is difficult to describe. We are unable to assess the value of the lost opportunity which would have occurred if the service had not been available. Because of this difficulty, consumers of services tend to rely on factors external to a specific product—such as reputation, ambience, appearance, friendliness, confidence, etc.

The degree of intangibility varies for different library products. All products have some intangible aspects and in fact most cannot be tried in advance. Therefore, although services are more intangible than goods, this alone may not be a key distinction. However, it is more important when tied to the people-intensive nature of services.

Services are perishable. Availability is limited by the number of personnel who can provide the service. We can't stockpile circulation desk assistants, bringing out five when we have a sudden influx of users, and storing them until they are needed again. Although some service organizations hire temporary personnel for unusually high-use periods, there is a limit to the ability of a service organization to match inventory with product demand.

Standardization of services is difficult. It is possible to define the services which will be available, but it isn't possible to specify what a given consumer will consider as the key determinant of quality, nor is it possible to control to any extent the performance of those providing the service. Since the person who provides the service is usually the key to pleasing the consumer of the service, there will be greater variability with services than with goods. "No matter how well-trained or motivated they might be, people make mistakes, forget, commit indiscretions, and at times are uncongenial. . . ." Further, "Unique to intangible products is the fact that the customer is seldom aware of being served well."[8]

CLIENT/CONSUMER

If libraries are to develop effective exchange relationships and maintain them on a permanent basis, then it is important to know who our potential consumers are, what they need, and which of these needs the library can meet. In order to do this, it is necessary to look at those who are consumers or potential consumers and divide them into groups who use certain products in a certain manner or who respond to distribution, promotion, and pricing criteria in a particular way.[9] Unfortunately, although this sounds logical on the surface, it is somewhat difficult to apply. The problem is trying to decide what is homogeneous about a given group of consumers other than their market behavior. It often appears that the segments which react in a certain way to market stimuli are perversely diverse in respect to all other criteria. In spite of the difficulty of being able to precisely define segment characteristics, it is helpful to look at these characteristics in order to be aware of the possible implications for market behavior.

There are a number of ways health science libraries can group users. Traditionally, these users have been described as students, basic science faculty, clinicians, researchers, etc.; that is, they have been described in terms of their primary occupation. They also can be classified by describing the benefits which they seek, because such a classification will help librarians describe product parameters (really the market offering characteristics) which are important to them.[10] Such parameters include acquiring ideas for new work; supporting work in progress, keeping current, developing competence; and preparing educational materials.[11]

Some of these activities require that the library produce an information product quickly, others require comprehensive coverage of the field, while still other activities might require that the product be available at a convenient location if it is to be used at all. For example, a clinician treating a patient for a specific disorder wants the most relevant and the most current information, and requires that information to be provided quickly. The same person teaching a class would want the same type of information, but might also desire information on the changes in therapeutic modalities which have occurred over the years. Also, he probably would have a more generous time frame in which to acquire that information.[10] Combining this approach with other consumer characteristics will divulge considerable information about the potential of a given segment as well as how libraries can best gain the full benefit of that potential. Buyer behavior characteristics which need to be examined include use-rate, loyalty, times of use, awareness of products, sensitivity to price, and sensitivity to quality.

Finally, although segmenting the library's market solely on the basis of demographics and geographic characteristics is not useful, it is important to consider the impact of such characteristics as age, profession, income, education, and location in relation to the information facility. Research projects which have examined the relationship between demographic and benefit variables in promotion have shown that a consideration of the combination of these two types of consumer characteristics enabled the marketer to develop the strongest package to reach a given market.[12]

ENVIRONMENTAL ANALYSIS

Although the consumer is the focus of the marketing program, the environment as a whole needs to be considered. A key aspect of the environment is the organizational environment which should be examined closely so that the library's contribution to the continuing existence and effective functioning of the organization can be defined. As Naisbitt has pointed out in *Megatrends,* this analysis of the institution's mission revolves around the answer to the question, "What business are you really in?"[13] Librarians, like many other specialists, have operated under the misconception that ". . .there's a divine dispensation that their markets are theirs—and no one else's. Yet no businessman in a free society can control a market when the customer decides to go elsewhere."[13] At the other extreme are those who are convinced that libraries and librarians are doomed to extinction; they are equally incorrect. Librarians must face the reality of living in a changing world. We do not have a divine right to the roles which we have filled, nor are we doomed to extinction. What is required is that we change with our environment. We need a vision about the business which we are in and that vision must be consistent with the world in which we live.

Stating our mission in generic terms is one way to recognize the role which libraries fill and to describe that role in a way which provides the library with the most flexibility in dealing with a changing environment. For example, first: "The role of the special library [is] achieving equal access to scientific information. . . ."[14] Secondly, the special library should, "Provide free access to, and promote the communication of, ideas and information so that individuals on their own behalf, and groups, agencies, organizations, and institutions can take active control of their lives and affairs."[15]

Computer centers are now beginning to call themselves information centers; libraries have been information centers for ages. However, too often they have been described in terms of what they have, not in terms of what they are designed to do.

In addition to defining the library's mission, it should be recognized that the library has many different competitors, both internal and external. There is competition for funding from other departments in the institution. The library competes for users of information services with departmental libraries, drug information centers, and user-friendly database vendors to mention only a few. If we are in competition with these other sources of information, we need to decide how we will compete. The primary basis for competition depends on the specific product, but includes quality, time, convenience, comprehensiveness, and price. For a given product, the basis for competition should be carefully assessed; if, for that product it is not possible to beat the competitor on the primary basis of competition, may want to consider seriously whether that product should continue to be offered.

MARKETING PROGRAM

The total market offering is a useful way to look at the goods and services provided by a library. Traditionally, products, distribution, promotion, and price are considered as separate, although coordinated, aspects of the marketing program. However, the total market offering concept recognizes that consumers do not clearly differentiate between these components of the exchange process. Since this seems to be particularly true for services, we will look at those factors which are relevant to the exchange process without attempting to dwell on their separateness.

Products

Products are often thought of as physical objects or activities which have value for buyers. As noted above, this definition unduly limits the description of the item purchased, because it simultaneously oversimplifies the concept and complicates the application of marketing theory. Instead, using the total marketing offering results in focusing on the total benefits and satisfactions which are desired by the consumer. Focusing activities on providing satisfactions means focusing on consumer needs, and this is necessary for a library if it is to remain a viable part of its institution or community. This activity requires defining the library's products in generic terms. For example, health sciences libraries often define their products in terms of specific product forms: books, audiovisuals, clinical librarians, LATCH, etc. However, if we resist the tendency to be myopic, then we know that we acquire, organize, manage, retrieve, and disseminate information. Libraries support educational, research, and patient care activities. If we do not think in terms of the benefits sought, we may offer a service for which there is no market, or we may not communicate accurately the product's benefits when we promote it. The problems which can occur for the library when this happens are obviously life-threatening.[16]

Describing the library's products in generic terms requires the definition of specific values which may accrue to users of the library's information products and criteria which the consumers consider important. One useful device for describing the values which consumers desire is the means-end chain theory, which attempts to explain the way "a person's selection of a service enables him or her to achieve his or her desired end state."[17] Desirable consequences may take the form of feeling comfortable, saving time and effort, or providing quality patient care. For example, convenience, timeliness, and reliability may be as much of the decision to use a product as the basic need for information. Undesirable consequences could include feeling dehumanized, annoyed, uncomfortable, or helpless.[17]

Although quality is a key criterion, it is difficult to define, because it is influenced both by the consumer and the supplier. Thus delivering a well-done search or producing an interlibrary loan in as expeditious a manner as possible is not enough. ". . .Managing service quality involves managing customer expectations and perceptions as well as the service assembly process."[18] In order to influence consumers' expectations and perceptions we must do more than ask the library's employees to do a good job, in the technical sense. We must identify what our consumers see as quality. Quality has been characterized as: price/value relationship, uniqueness, and expectations exceeded,[18] or as ". . .doing consistently well those hundreds—even thousands—of little things that satisfy our customers. . . ."[19] Particularly important, then, is defining what a consumer expects and then exceeding that expectation on a regular basis.

Quality assessment must be facilitated by establishing reasonable levels of expected performance which can be used to judge the quality of the service rendered. Services need to be made tangible in order to guide the consumer to find those services that he wants, to educate him about alternative services and finally, to teach him about the uniqueness of the service.[20]

Because of the relative intangible nature of "service," the consumer often lacks a concrete set of product expectations upon which to base his/her satisfaction. This is further complicated by the simultaneous production and delivery of the product. Research has shown that everyone has a set of expectations about the typical characteristics expected in regard to what events will occur in a given situation, who will be involved, and the setting in which these events will occur. These expectations serve as the basis for judging satisfaction, especially in service situations where product expectations are often nebulous. By developing a script for a service encounter, a basis for evaluation can be provided; if there are deviations from what is expected then satisfaction will be affected.[21]

Furthermore, the script will provide a basis for promotion of the service. By identifying what is expected by clients, what they perceive as important, we can address these concerns in our promotion. That is, we can reassure our clients that their expectations will be met or exceeded, thereby reducing the risk which they may associate with making a decision about the use of a service. Further, these expectations can be given attention in our daily interactions with library users.

Of course, it is neither necessary nor possible for every user's preconceptions about library services to be met, but we need to know what most of our library's users expect. For example, the expectations of undergraduate nursing students about the type of facility, appearance and demeanor of personnel, and the conduct of other users materially differs from those of a research professor in biochemistry. While we cannot vary all parameters to meet these differing expectations, we need to be aware of those events which if they occur will result in a negative disconfirmation for that client, and we need to minimize the impact of such events. At the same time, those events which will be negative for all types of users should be identified, that is, those experiences that will fall consistently below their expectations. For example, unfriendly, unhelpful, or less than competent personnel, who fail to produce a product by a promised delivery time, or who fail to have available those items needed for accessing a product fully, will provide negative experiences for all users.

Finally, as noted earlier, a particular problem with intangibles is that consumers are not aware of quality until it is lacking. That is, negative discontinuance is more likely to be noted than positive discontinuance. Further, small visible failures are often seen as the tip of the iceberg. Therefore, it is necessary on a regular basis to remind clients of what they are getting so that small failures will not be so glaring and so likely to be seen more readily and more important than the quality products which they receive regularly.[8]

The importance of all public contact personnel should be recognized, since they need to be sensitive to their key role in customer satisfaction. The number of people with whom a user must interact to obtain a service should be minimized, because the employee is often a surrogate for the service, and it is necessary to manage the employer/client interactions to elicit positive consumer participation and to generate a "pleasant, satisfying service purchase experience" for the long term.[20]

The interaction of supplier and client, an integral part of the service experience which may be highly emotional, adds to the possibility of disconfirmation of expectations. If a consumer has to wait too long at a service point, especially when he/she expected rapid service, then anger results. Therefore, often a consumer's decision about a service provider's potential for delivering a satisfactory product is related to his/her expectation about the probable emotional outcome of the experience. The evaluation of all the separate aspects at a cognitive level, knowing what will be provided, is not adequate. The library user may not be convinced solely by being told the kind of information which will be provided by an online search or by the type of instruction which the library can provide for students. Rather the decision about whether to use these services may be based on the anticipated overall effect of using the service. Therefore, promotional efforts should be aimed at stimulating "feelings" which would meet the potential consumer's expectations.[22]

Distribution

In order for a product to be used the consumer must obtain it. For services this often presents special problems, because often the producer of the service must be available when it is consumed. The reference librarian looks up the answer to a question and almost simultaneously transmits it to the user. Barriers to distribution are spatial, temporal, physical, and perceptual. Any one or all four of these barriers may be present at any given time. The clinical librarian and LATCH programs are examples of efforts to overcome spatial and temporal barriers by taking the service provider and the information product out to users. Telecommunications and computer technology have provided new means for removing barriers which are the result of being separated in time and space from potential consumers.

Perceptual barriers are often overlooked. The image of the library may discourage use. All too often we hear: "You **never** have anything I want," or, "The library is **so slow.**" Such judgments may not be accurate, but they affect the consumption of library products. Perceptual barriers can be created by the appearance and arrangement of the library, the dress and demeanor of the personnel, and even the appearance and conduct of other clients.

Furthermore, research has shown that service providers' perceptions of factors which influence the choice of a provider are significantly different from those factors which consumers of that service see as important. One research study found that consumers of marketing research services felt that the most important factor in selecting a vendor of those services was the usefulness of the research produced by that vendor; the other two concerns in selecting a service provider were the quality of the research and how well the firm understood the client's problems. The marketing research firms indicated that they perceived the firm's reputation as the most important factor used by consumers when they were making purchase decisions. The quality of the research and referral by satisfied customers were seen as the second and third most important criteria. Both groups ranked advertising as the least important factor, and the clients ranked price as seventh of ten factors.[23] Librarians need to be aware of these differences in perceptions about what is relevant in the choice of a supplier. While our clients may not have a readily available alternative supplier of information services, they may decide not to be a consumer of library information services at all. Further, when library services are promoted, it is necessary to focus on the factors which the potential consumers perceive as influential in their selection of a service provider.

Promotion

Although promotion is interwoven with products in a service organization, it is still necessary to develop specific promotional activities. Promotion involves "all the tools whose major purpose is persuasive communication, that is the communicator consciously arranges the message and selects the channel to have a calculated effect on the attitude or behavior of a specific audience."[24] Promotion includes advertising and publicity as well as a number of other devices used by libraries to publicize their products and services such as annual reports, bulletin boards, brochures, memoranda, speaking engagements, and every contact with a user.

In designing promotional messages, regardless of the specific format, it is important to keep in mind the basic communication model: **who** says **what** to **whom** through what **chan-**

nel? In every case the intended audience should be the key determinant of the other components of the message. There are a number of considerations which can serve as guides in the development of promotional materials. The competitive framework in which the library exists is one such consideration. What other services and products are competing with us? Further, are these very similar, or are they somewhat different products designed to meet the same need? That is, are we competing with another library (very similar) or with an information broker (somewhat different); this approach enables the library to see its competitive edge which can be emphasized in promotional efforts.

Promotional messages should implicitly answer many of the key questions which a consumer might ask about the service organization. The library's world should be created in the mind of the client. The promotional material should indicate the scope of the library's activities including what makes these activities special. Many people think of library use as slow, laborious, and time-consuming. We want them to see the library as providing quick, trouble-free, reliable service.

Promotional messages should create an appropriate personality for the library. Over time, clients should come to see the library as someone with whom they are familiar, whom they trust, and for whom they have the highest regard. The library should be clearly identified with meeting the client's needs. We want to project an image of ourselves and our services that appeals to and compliments our primary audience's needs, values, life styles, and attitudes. The library should be seen as an integral part of the life of the organization. Promotional messages should lead clients to the library.[25]

Services can be designed to satisfy users' important information needs, but if our clients do not know about them or do not understand how such services will help them, then they can not and will not use them.

Price

Until a few years ago, most librarians believed that price was an irrelevant concept because libraries did not charge for many of their services. Although the advent of online searching, interlibrary loan fees, and coin-operated photocopy machines has made more librarians aware of price concerns, many are not fully aware of the implications which cost concepts hold for library operations. Price is usually thought of in terms of monetary cost rather than in relation to all of its components. There are several types of costs associated with accessing a service. These costs are money, time, effort, and psyche.[26]

Generally, librarians have been most concerned with the implications which fee-based services have for access to those services. As pricing theory indicates, there is an assumption that as costs increase, use decreases.[27] However, not much attention has been given to the implications for access of other prices which the user must pay for library services. Adam Smith indicated, "The real price of everything, what everything really costs to the man who wants to acquire it, is the toil and trouble of acquiring it." In each case, money, time, effort, and psyche may represent a cost or a benefit which are a component in the total price paid for a service. Further, as one cost increases, another may decrease. The use of computerized searching services may reduce the costs of time and effort associated with accessing information, while at the same time, the out-of-pocket monetary costs may be greater than when the client expended his/her own time and effort. Of course, the time and effort costs are not reduced to zero, since the consumer cannot just think of the topic on which information is needed and have it magically appear instantaneously. Further, there are psychic costs involved. Psychic costs include self-esteem, pride, privacy, control, and freedom from risk, etc. Using library services may reduce or increase such costs. To request an interlibrary loan or to ask a librarian for assistance in locating a book on a topic is to pay a price for reduced privacy. Code of ethics notwithstanding, who among us wants our name on the interlibrary loan form for "Living with Herpes"? Also, there are costs associated with self-esteem and pride. Sometimes the product received increases self-esteem, pride, and peace of mind. Yet to ask for information results in a cost to the user. The less secure a person is the more likely the cost will be too high.

CONCLUSION

In order for marketing to be utilized in library public service activities, librarians need to be aware of the basic theoretical concepts which define marketing and of the unique challenges presented because of the intangible, consumer-intensive nature of library activities. However, it is equally important to recognize that these traits require that all personnel be motivated and customer-conscious.[28] Employees must realize the importance of their role as part of the product, promotion, price, and distribution of the product or service. It is not enough to be technically competent. It is equally important for employees to be steeped in the image of the organization and to adopt the service/client orientation as their own. This orientation is as important for technical service personnel as it is for those in public services.

REFERENCES

1. Lynn, R.A. *Marketing: Principles and Market Actions.* New York: McGraw Hill, 1969.

2. Holloway, R.J., and Hancock, R.S. *Marketing in a Changing Environment.* New York: John Wiley & Sons, 1973.

3. Ford, Neil M. et al. "Introducing Marketing into Service Organizations: A Case Study." In: Leonard L. Barry, G. Lynn Shostack, and Gregory D. Upah, eds. *Emerging Perspectives on Services Marketing.* Chicago: American Marketing Association, 1983, pp. 120–123.

4. Kotler, Philip. *Marketing Management.* 4th ed. Englewood Cliffs: Prentice Hall, 1980.

5. Brown, James R., and Fern, Edward. "Goods vs. Services Marketing: A Divergent Perspective." In: James H. Donnelly and William R. George, eds. *Marketing of Services.* Chicago: American Marketing Association, 1981, pp. 205–207.

6. Lovelock, Christopher H. "Think Before You Leap in Services Marketing." In: *Emerging Perspectives on Services Marketing,* pp. 115–119.

7. Thomas, Dan R.E. "Strategy is Different in Service Business." *Harvard Business Review* 78 (July/August 1978): 158–165.

8. Levitt, Theodore. "Marketing Intangible Products and Product Intangibles." *Harvard Business Review* 81 (May/June 1981): 94–102.

9. Levy, Sidney J. *Marketplace Behavior.* New York: AMACOM, 1978.

10. Ferguson, Douglas. "Marketing Online Services in the University." *Online* 1 (July 1977): 15–23.

11. Back, Harry. "What Information Dissemination Studies Imply Concerning the Design of On-line Reference Retrieval Systems." *Journal of the American Society for Information Science* 23 (May/June 1972): 156–163.

12. Lewis, Robert C. "Marketing for Full Service Restaurants—An Analysis of Demographic and Benefit Segmentation." In: *Marketing of Services,* pp. 43–46.

13. Naisbitt, John. *Megatrends*. New York: Warner Books, 1982, p. 86.

14. Hubbard, William. "Closing the Gap: Understanding Utilization." In: Compiled by Pamela Jones and Marcy Murphy. *Issues and Involvement*. New York: Special Library Association, 1983.

15. Public Library Principles Task Force. Public Library Association. "The Public Library: Democracy's Resource." Cited in *Library Journal* 108 (January 1, 1983): 5.

16. Davis, Duane L., and Joyce, Mary L. "Product Development in Nonprofit Service Organizations." In: Ronald D. Taylor, John H. Summey, and Blaise J. Bergiel, eds. *Progress in Marketing Theory and Practice*. Carbondale, Ill.: Southern Marketing Association, 1981, pp. 25–28.

17. Gutman, Johnathan and Reynolds, Thomas J. "Developing Images for Services through Means-End Chain Analysis." In: *Emerging Perspectives on Services Marketing*, pp. 40–44.

18. Lewis, Robert C., and Booms, Bernard H. "The Marketing Aspects of Service Quality." In *Emerging Perspectives on Services Marketing*, pp. 99–100.

19. Crosby, William E. "Remarks." In: *Emerging Perspectives on Services Marketing*, pp. 100–102.

20. George, William R.; Kelly, Patrick J.; and Marshall, Claudia E. "Personal Selling of Services." In: *Emerging Perspectives on Services Marketing*, pp. 65–67.

21. Smith, Ruth A., and Houston Michael J. "Script-Based Evaluations of Satisfaction with Services." In: *Emerging Perspectives on Services Marketing*, pp. 59–61.

22. Young, Robert F. "The Advertising of Consumer Services and the Hierarchy of Effects." In: *Marketing of Services*, pp. 196–199.

23. Parasuraman, A., and Zeithaml, Valarie A. "Differential Perspectives of Suppliers and Clients of Industrial Services." In: *Emerging Perspectives on Services Marketing*, pp. 35–39.

24. Kotler, Philip. *Marketing for Nonprofit Organizations*. Englewood Cliffs: Prentice Hall, 1975.

25. Firestone, Sidney J. "Why Advertising a Service is Different." In: *Emerging Perspectives on Service Marketing*, pp. 86–89.

26. Fine, Seymour H. "Beyond Money: The Concept of Social Price." In: *Marketing of Services*, pp. 113–115.

27. Huston, Mary M. "Fee or Free." *Library Journal* 104 (September 15, 1979): 1811–1814.

28. Gronroos, Christian. "Internal Marketing—An Integral Part of Marketing Theory." In: *Marketing of Services*, pp. 236–238.

Marketing Information Services Outside the Medical Center

Henry L. Lemkau, Jr.
Suzetta Burrows
August La Rocco

ABSTRACT. Most academic health sciences libraries conduct outreach programs, but few market information services outside the medical center. This paper examines the steps necessary for the development of a marketing program. The elements of the marketing process itself are applied to a library's vending information services. Described are the impact of marketing information services on the library and methods to determine its success. Economic changes during the first four years of the eighties will cause an exponential increase in marketing activity by health sciences libraries of all types.

INTRODUCTION

The age of innocence for health sciences libraries is passing into history. Deep cuts in federal support of higher education and research and the implementation of DRGs (Diagnosis Related Groups) as the method of compensation for most of the nation's hospitals during the first four years of the eighties are causing competition for the health care dollar to become

Henry Lemkau is Director and Chairman, Department of the Library and Biomedical Communications; Suzetta Burrows is Vice-Chairman and Associate Director for Media and Regional Programs; and August La Rocco is Special Projects Librarian, at the Louis Calder Memorial Library, University of Miami School of Medicine, P.O. Box 016950, Miami, FL 33101.
Mr. Lemkau received his B. A. in history from St. John's University and his M. L. S. from Pratt Institute Graduate School of Library and Information Science.
Ms. Burrows received her B. S. in biology from Brooklyn College of the City University of New York and her M. L. S. from Columbia University School of Library Service.
Mr. La Rocco received his B. A. in psychology from New York University and his M. L. S. from Pratt Institute Graduate School of Library and Information Science.

143

progressively acute. With increasing frequency, educational institutions and health care facilities are looking beyond their walls for nontraditional support. For academic as well as non-academic health sciences libraries, these trends will see a more widespread marketing effort of information services of all types to many new and diverse constituencies.

Most academic health sciences libraries have been involved in outreach programs since the beginning of the National Library of Medicine's Regional Medical Library Program in the late sixties. Outreach services, although fee-based in recent years, are provided in most cases for a nominal charge designed to recover direct costs. Indirect costs, which can be higher than direct costs, are either partially or totally supported by the library. The library views the community as a homogeneous group; consequently its outreach services are offered for standard fees, on a first-come, first-served basis. The library attempts to keep pace with existing demand, and makes no attempt to stimulate demand for its outreach services. .

Deans of medical schools and administrators of hospitals are now, however, mandating that libraries become income-producing and designating a specific service or product in some cases. "Outreach," the catchword of the seventies, is being replaced in the eighties with "entrepreneurial." Direct cost recovery is being supplanted by the cost plus philosophy. As a result, town and gown are no longer insular universes set apart by an ivy barrier.

The first four years of the eighties also are marked by the microcomputer revolution and America's transformation from an industrial, product-oriented to an informational, service-oriented economy.[1] Librarians' long history of computer literacy, expertise in information retrieval, experience with in-house and outreach activities and strong service orientation, place them in an excellent position to comply with new mandates. All that is needed is a reaffirmation of information's tremendous value to all sectors of the community and an understanding of the marketing process.

Information can easily be regarded as a product having intrinsic value. Thus, its transfer to a consumer at an established price is a marketing transaction and the community becomes the marketplace. This calls into play elements of the marketing process. The process sets organizational goals, delineates strategies and policies to attain these goals, and develops plans to assure that the strategies are successfully implemented. This paper examines the preliminary steps in developing a marketing program and the elements of the entire process itself. Throughout, marketing the computer search services of an academic health sciences library serves as the model.

ORGANIZATIONAL GOALS AND STRUCTURE

To market effectively, administration must first establish marketing as a primary goal for the library. Ideally, the library's parent institution, its school and university or its hospital, should have this as an institutional goal as well. In this case, the library is again reflecting the goals of its institution and there is an existing institutional structure to coordinate with and rely upon. Close ties should be formed between the library and the individual responsible for the institution's community affairs. Contributions of significant sums, $1,000 or more, are appropriately recognized by the library director, as well as by the dean of the school and president of the university or the administrator of the hospital. In some cases, the institution's administrators might lend their names to promotional materials as well. Fee structures developed should be consistent with those of the parent institution and contracts entered into should be approved by the institution's legal counsel and have institutional support.

Internally, an individual able to commit and speak for the library should be designated as head of the marketing effort. This person's name and business card should accompany all materials relating to the effort and all queries should be referred to this individual. If there is a marketing committee, this person should serve as its chair. In the absence of a marketing committee, a mechanism to accommodate staff input and the many changes resulting from the marketing effort should be established. Since frequent consultation with the library director and a support staff are essential, the individual responsible for marketing should be in the administrative office. Needless to say, this individual should have proven oral, written and interpersonal skills.

EXISTING LIBRARY SERVICES AND MARKETS

Marketing presupposes more than a cursory knowledge of the marketplace, i.e., the community. One must learn what the marketplace consists of and what it expects. One must also understand that there is no one market, but a diversity of markets in every community, that is, clusters of individuals and institutions, each cluster with differing needs and expectations. This is known as market segmentation. The concept of segmentation is fundamental to successful marketing. It directs the marketer to view the market not as a mass of buyers with essentially similar needs, but as a set of sub-groups, each of which commands a separate strategy.[2]

Prior to developing a marketing program, an inventory and evaluation of the library's existing services and various market segments should be conducted. Lists of services currently rendered and of the individuals and institutions currently served outside the medical center should be made. The revenue derived from each of these services and from each segment of the market should be identified. The library's strengths and weaknesses in each segment of the market should be evaluated with respect to the needs of each segment and the availability of competing services. How the market's needs interact with the library's ability to meet them, versus the ability of others, must be addressed.

As an example, an academic health sciences library might typically provide computerized searches to a community not affiliated with the medical center. That community might be representative of (1) primary health care professionals who request searches directly or through an intermediary at another institution without access to these databases; (2) attorneys, with access to the LEXIS and/or Westlaw databases but no others; and (3) corporate individuals, such as chemists and pharmacologists at pharmaceutical firms with either inadequate or no library facilities. After identification, the library determines the current size of each existing market segment by calculating the number of searches done for and/or the income derived from each. The current size is an excellent indicator of the existing need for the service.

The comprehensiveness of the library service and the expertise and efficiency of the staff responsible for the service are determined by comparing them with other sources of these services available to the market. Commercial services such as the EMPIRES component of the AMA/NET service, those available from information brokers and end user searching services, as well as comparable services offered by other libraries in the area, are identified and studied for comparative purposes. How does the EMPIRES component compare with MEDLINE in terms of marketing strength: scope of database, access points, document delivery service, etc? What are the educational backgrounds, database training qualifications, and expertise of the searchers of these other services? What are their fees, volume, turnaround time, and promotional strategies? What other services are offered? In short, how do the quality, quantity and price of competing services compare to those being considered for marketing?

Competition exists for most library services. Discovery and continuous study of competing services are essential to identify the library's current and future strengths and weaknesses. Information about competing services is also highly useful to subsequent pricing and promotional aspects of the marketing process.

The current workload of existing staff should be assessed at this time. To market a service successfully, trained staff must be available to perform the additional workload generated by the successful marketing of the service. This might necessitate a shift of existing staff and duties, training, and/or an increase in levels of staffing. If the second phase of developing a market program, that is, identifying the need, is done properly, an increase in staff can be justified. Frequently, the old adage applies: you have to spend money to make money. Administrators at institutions are well aware of this and more willing to approve increased expenditures if the projected increases in revenue offset them.

MARKET ANALYSIS

Marketing programs must not be designed from preconceptions of what a monolithic public wants, but from a systematic inquiry into the knowledge, attitude, and practice of a diverse populace.[3] This dictates that the health sciences library adopt a marketing posture, the key dimensions of which are pointed up by Shapiro:

1. Willingness to take one's marching orders from the market
2. Commitment to making the library a responsive organization
3. Recognition that some products may have outlived their usefulness and substituted for new offerings.[4]

Taking one's marching orders from the market presupposes a study and a determination of its needs in measurable terms. It should be stressed that the heart of marketing is the design of products or services for the requirements of separate groups. Having identified these needs, the library should then determine how well they are being satisfied before any effort is undertaken to fill them.[5] It may be that a market segment relies on other sources or services, in which case a marketing program cannot be justified unless the product to be marketed is demonstrably superior.

A study of the characteristics of the community should include the influences which shape it. These include environmental factors such as demographic, environmental and sociological trends, all of which may influence demand. Sources of market information are of two types, primary and secondary. Primary data are derived from field surveys in which participants respond to questionnaires, and personal or telephone interviews. It is important that field research be aimed at those who are responsible for decision making. Secondary data are obtained from internal records, such as annual reports, or published sources, such as government statistics, association publications, area directories, almanacs, etc.

Continuing the example of computer searches, the community's need for and all sources of this service must be determined. Primary data on the searching services at area health care facilities and corporations can be gathered by questionnaires or telephone calls to administrators responsible for library services. Lists of institutions with MEDLINE services or directories of services offered and clientele served by area libraries are secondary sources of this information. The percentage of health care institutions in the area with these services can be determined by identifying all area institutions from the yellow pages under "hospitals," the American Hospital Association *Guide to the Health Care Field,* and directories of state or area hospital associations.

As a point of reference, only twenty-five of the one hundred health care facilities in the geographic area served by the institution with which the authors are affiliated have a library, and not all of these libraries have computer search services. Of those libraries that do have these services, none routinely does searches for individuals unaffiliated with their institution, although they are frequently asked. Lawyers are frequent requesters at these area libraries and at the academic health sciences library. The number of individuals listed in the yellow pages under "attorneys-trial-practice-personal injury & wrongful death" is substantial. There are also numerous listings under "associations," "clinics-medical," "health maintenance organizations," "laboratories-medical," "pharmaceutical products," etc., for organizations and corporations with health information needs and no library.

Demographic projections indicate a continuous increase in the area's already diverse populations. Many of the area's hospitals without libraries are now corporately owned, and there is little evidence of professional hospital library development at these institutions. Similarly, the area is attracting new industry without library facilities. The community's need for these services is further illustrated by the availability of comparable services for the health sciences community from the local state university library, the main branch of the public library in a neighboring county, by a pharmaceutical house for promotional purposes, and from several commercial information brokers.

MARKETING STANCE AND MARKET PERCEPTION

The needs addressed by the library and the future of each segment of the library's market should also be determined. These determinations form the library's philosophy or vision which will be exhibited in its marketing stance. The market's current perception of the library and its institution should be determined as well. Factors viewed by the market include the policies, personnel, technical excellence, reputation for accuracy and dependability, pricing, and professionalism of the library and its institution. Its image, therefore, springs from the actual performance of the organization. The library's marketing stance should address any changes in the market's current perception deemed necessary to create an image of excellence. As Kotler astutely observes, "It is the organization's image, not necessarily the reality, that people respond to."[6] Its stance also will greatly affect the market's future perception of the library and its institution which, in turn, will impact the marketing effort.

Having established in the previous market analysis step that there is a need in the community for computerized searches of the literature, the specific needs addressed by the services are now identified. For example, the practicing physician needs these services to quickly identify current, relevant, and reliable information for patient care decisions. The corporate scientist needs these same services to be comprehensive for research and development activities. Attorneys require that these services identify highly specific information and sometimes general background information as well. One must recognize the likelihood that each of these market segments will continue to rely on automated information retrieval and demand improvements as they become available and are marketed by database vendors and producers, equipment and communications firms.

Various market segments recognize the library's vision when it exhibits knowledge of these specific needs in its marketing stance. The library projects technically excellent, accurate, dependable, responsive and state-of-the-art search services by qualified, trained, service-oriented librarians. If the potential market's current perception of the library differs, as determined by questionnaires, personal interviews and conversations with recent recipients of its services, this new stance must be specifically addressed in-house and then in the marketing process.

PLANNING

Having identified and described a market segment(s) and developed a marketing stance to meet a determined need, the library must now decide whether or not to market. Based upon a favorable perception of the library's expertise and service and the assumption that the preliminary steps indicate marketing is justified, the library must then design a well-defined plan, which it will publicize and distribute. The bottom line to successful marketing is careful planning.

The first step in the planning process is to list the ideas and concepts generated in the preliminary marketing steps. The second is to subject this conceptualization to a screening process. Estimate the demand from each market segment for each service to be marketed and the potential revenue from each based on several pricing algorithms. When pricing a service, a moderate position based on a balanced assessment of market needs and the ability of the library to respond to these needs is recommended. Consider the suitability of marketing each service to each segment of the existing market, the ability of the library to meet the estimated demand, and the "fit" of the product and of the market segment with the vision of the library. Now, develop a preliminary plan. Submit it to library administration and/or the institution's administration. Get the approval of the institution's legal counsel and the support of the library committee, the institution and its community affairs representative.

Set reasonable objectives and plan the promotion campaign around these objectives. Objectives should be expressed in quantitative terms and a time frame for achieving them should be established. For example, an objective may be to increase the number of searches done for attorneys by 25 percent within a year. It is important that not too many objectives be set at once. It also is important that decisions regarding objectives be shared with the staff. This will tend to make the objectives more realistic and it will motivate the staff to attain them. Continue to revise the plan based on feedback and changes in the information arena and then promote these new or improved services.

The original plan and pricing rationale of the library with which the authors are affiliated has been previously described elsewhere.[7] Although the example to date has been computer searches, the decision was made in the original plan to market all information services of the Department of the Library and Biomedical Communications to the surrounding ten county area with existing staff. Services are offered on a "cost plus" basis to all professionals with a health information need on both an individual and a subscription basis. The fee structure developed reflects various market segments. The institution's indirect cost factor for government sponsored research, the fees of competing services, and maximum fees for services set by the National Library of Medicine and individual regions were the pricing guidelines. The promotional campaign regulated the demand, even though too many objectives were set at once. The subscription plan was publicized initially to health care institutions, but promotion to other market segments continued over an eighteen-month period. Some services were not promoted until the third year because it was anticipated that the demand would exceed the Library's ability to meet it.

Once a marketing plan is in place, it must be continuously revised based on user response and demand. The library's awareness of possible improvements and new developments in the information arena also necessitate constant revision. A problem with the original subscription plan with which the authors have experience was underutilization of services by member institutions. Indeed, one institution did not renew their subscription for this reason. The implementation of a circuit rider program for member institutions is an example of plan enhancement and revision. In this program, a Library faculty member visits the member institution one-half day each week. The librarian provides computer searches on site and on demand and arranges for document delivery and other services available with the institution's membership. The librarian visits departments of the member institution and provides other outreach services to them, such as photocopies of the title pages of the journal issues received at the member institution that week. As such, the circuit rider is not only visible evidence that the institution is indeed providing information services to its staff and employees, but is integral to maintaining and increasing the volume of services requested.

Currently in the planning stages is the use of electronic mail to "upload" the results of computer searches done on a microcomputer to a remote requester the same day. This capability has been demanded by an institution prior to their joining the Library as a member. This service will be available only to member institutions and typifies the general trend of the Library to encourage institutions to use the services being marketed on a subscription, rather than on an individual basis.

An element of the original plan that has not changed is marketing services to the community with existing staff. With the increased workload that has resulted from the marketing effort, adhering to this element has dictated the establishment of a true priority basis for members for all services. It also dictates that should an institution require circuit rider services more than one-half day each week, the institution will need to hire a librarian. Setting limits on services or on user demands is necessary in a successful marketing effort. Seeking new market segments is also important to its success. Examples could include the development of consumer health information services for the institution's lay constituency.

PROMOTION

The author's experience with the circuit rider services also points to the importance of continuous promotion of information services. Although the need for a service can be clearly indicated in the market analysis step, need does not always translate into demand. A recent study by the National Academy of Sciences is an excellent case in point.[8] Two-way home video education to achieve a high school equivalancy diploma was offered in Sparternburg, S. C. where 62 percent of the population had not completed high school. While there was a true need, only a disappointing percentage of the population availed themselves of the service. Clearly, need did not equate with desire. In the promotion aspects of the marketing process, therefore, it is not enough to simply announce a new service. Desire for a service must be stimulated as well. With information services, stimulating desire must be a continuous process. With all services, the scope and frequency of the promotional campaign should be geared to the accomplishments of objectives set in the planning process.

Promoting services can be accomplished through various channels. All United States consumers and practicing professionals are well aware of these channels: direct mail, space advertisement, media releases and spots, publications, exhibits and demonstrations. Direct mail is a common first channel for marketing information services. A brochure can be made and mailed with letters aimed at the various market segments. The brochure can describe the service as a whole; the letter should be addressed to each market segment, stimulating its desire and demonstrating that the service is the best possible solution. Purchasing mailing labels from the membership lists of various associations or from a commercial house will greatly facilitate bulk mailings of this kind. In terms of realizing objectives, a three percent to five percent return in a direct mail campaign is considered good.

Space advertisement also is recommended in the membership directories of professional associations in the community and in their journals, newsletters and other publications. Articles written specifically for these publications are even more effective and therefore highly recommended. As with all promotional materials, articles should speak to a specific market segment and include information gathered prior to the development of the marketing program. Current topics of interest, such as information applications of computer technology, are of broad enough appeal to appear in local newspapers, general community magazines, and on local television programs.

Exhibits at professional meetings held in the area and demonstrations at these meetings and at professional staff meetings in the community are particularly effective. Both exhibits and demonstrations permit personal communication, the single most effective method of announcing the advantages of a service and stimulating desire for it. Applicable in both are promotional pieces such as brochures, posters, and video or slide/tape productions on the services being marketed. In the authors' experience, a direct mail campaign aimed solely at arranging a personal meeting was very successful in reaching hospital administrators, chiefs of staff and chairmen of medical education committees. A tickler letter was sent to these individuals at hospitals known not to have a library, asking that the Library be called for a free evaluation of the institution's information services and information on cost-effective alternatives to developing a full library facility on-site.

A newsletter or regular publication from the library to the market is also an effective promotional strategy. It is a good vehicle to announce not only the original plan but changes and improvements to it, positive effects of the marketing effort on the library and the market, and yardsticks of its success. Mailing this publication to individuals in the library's school or hospital serves as a constant reminder of the library's marketing efforts and makes individuals aware of services available to the community. In the daily lives of these practicing health professionals, they interact with colleagues in the community and can function most effectively as a personal promoter of the services.

DISTRIBUTION OF SERVICES

The final step in the marketing process is the distribution of services. Assuming the services being marketed also are offered in-house to the library's primary clientele, it is essential that the staff distribute services to both markets in the same way whenever possible. For example, the policies and procedures for circuit riders should be as consistent as possible with those for clinical librarians. Just as there is a mechanism for solving problems that result from the distribution of services within the medical center, there should be a mechanism, perhaps a hotline, for problems arising from the distribution of marketed services and for rush requests outside the medical center.

One must address a primary difference between in-house and out-of-house services, namely, the geographical distance of the requester from the library. The feasibility of a toll-free number should be investigated as a remedy to this problem for distant patrons. A messenger or delivery service to member institutions is highly recommended as a means of approximating the rapid transfer of information possible for in-house services. Circuit riders also can serve as messengers and requests for services should be filled by the time of their next visit. Electronic mail and facsimile transmission take on a new urgency when a library is marketing services to the community.

CONCLUSION

The decision to begin marketing information services outside the library, in general, makes it necessary to rethink what a library is and whom it serves. In the current information age, health sciences libraries are an integral part of the community. Libraries draw upon a multitude of information sources from networks and computerized databases throughout the local, regional and national arenas. In a reciprocal relationship, diverse segments of these communities call upon libraries for needed information. To develop a market program and work through the marketing process is to delineate the community and redefine the library. The library's role as a passive repository activated only upon request is transformed into an assertive, dynamic role, in which the library stimulates desire for its services and delivers these services in ways that impart their intrinsic value. Indeed, the library can actively develop new avenues for furthering its institution's goals in the process.

Initially, the success of the marketing effort should be measured by the ability of the information product to pay for itself and by the presence of an expanding market. Ultimately, it should be measured by the percentage of the library's budget that derives from the net income of marketed services, and by its impact on the degree of professional staff development, the strengthening of library resources, the development of new roles and services, and, perhaps most importantly, the visibility of the library both within and outside of its institution.

REFERENCES

1. Naisbitt, John. *Megatrends; Ten New Directions Transforming Our Lives.* New York: Warner Books, 1984, p.11.

2. Andreasen, Alan R. "Advancing Library Marketing." *Journal of Library Administration* 1 (Fall 1980): 17–32.

3. Sciandra, Russell C., and Stein, Judith A. "Applying Marketing Techniques to Promotion of the Cancer Information Service." *Progress in Clinical and Biological Research* 130 (1983): 153–160.

4. Shapiro, Stanley J. "Marketing and the Information Professional." *Special Libraries* 71 (November 1980): 469–74.

5. Bellardo, Trudi, and Waldart, Thomas J. "Marketing Products and Services in Academic Libraries." *Libri* 27 (September 1977):181–94.

6. Kotler, Philip. *Marketing for Nonprofit Organizations.* Englewood Cliffs, NJ: Prentice-Hall, Inc., 1975, pp. 129–130.

7. Burrows, Suzetta, and La Rocco, August. "Fees for Automated Reference Services in Academic Health Sciences Libraries: No Free Lunches." *Medical Reference Services Quarterly* 2 (Summer 1983): 1–11.

8. *Telecommunications for Metropolitan Areas: Opportunities for the 1980's.* A

Report by the Steering Committee for the Metropolitan Communications Study of the Board on Telecommunications-Computer Applications, Assembly of Engineering. National Research Council. Washington, D.C.: National Academy of Sciences, 1978, pp. 17–18.

The Marketing of Biomedical Information Service at the University of Minnesota: Creative Error Correction

Joan K. Freeman
Kathie A. O'Connell

ABSTRACT. Biomedical Information Service, the fee-based unit of the University of Minnesota's Bio-Medical Library, has moved from selling the service to marketing it. The processes involved in the change and the resulting effects are addressed within the framework of the "four P's" of marketing—product, price, place (i.e., distribution), and promotion. The examples cited stress the pragmatic application of marketing theory in the daily operation of this client-supported service.

INTRODUCTION

The phone call came in at eight a.m. A physician in North Dakota was preparing to perform a complex surgical procedure that afternoon. He needed to read a specific article on the surgical procedure before performing the operation. The University of Minnesota's Bio-Medical Library was the only library in the region that owned the journal. Could he get a copy of the article in time?

An attorney in a neighboring state needed to find the current locations of two physicians. The last available location on

Joan K. Freeman heads the marketing and public relations section of Biomedical Information Service. Kathie A. O'Connell is the head of Biomedical Information Service, Bio-Medical Library, University of Minnesota, 305 Diehl Hall, 505 Essex Street Southeast, Minneapolis, MN 55455. The authors gratefully acknowledge the contributions made by the entire staff of the University of Minnesota's Bio-Medical Library. The authors also wish to thank all the clients of Biomedical Information Service for their ongoing support and patronage.

either person was valid in 1971. Could Biomedical Information Service find this information quickly?

A man called in search of an article purported to be in the latest issue of a renowned medical journal. The article allegedly touted a new pill that suppressed snoring. This man wanted to know the name of the drug–or rather, his wife did. Could Biomedical Information Service help?

The above synopses are indicative of the types of client requests received by Biomedical Information Service, the fee-based unit of the University of Minnesota's Bio-Medical Library. The successful completion of these client requests reflects the marketing efforts which have been expended in behalf of this service. It is the intent of this article to provide examples of how marketing techniques have been utilized to improve Biomedical Information Service by making it more client sensitive. It is hoped that the experiences discussed herein will provide informational data which will supplement existing library marketing literature. The majority of the available literature discusses the theory involved in marketing a fee-based information service in a publicly supported academic library, but does not address the pragmatic application of that theory. This lack results perhaps from the proprietary nature of the information involved. This writing will forego the usual proprietary nature of this service and share the experience. of creatively correcting the errors made. Perhaps the largest error was believing that marketing and selling were one in the same.

Marketing and selling are two different concepts. Marketing begins and ends with the consumer. Its basic objective is to establish and maintain a mutually satisfying relationship between the consumer and the producer.[1] Selling, on the other hand, takes as its focal point the producer, and that producer's need to convert his or her product into cash.[2] Marketing is the process of customizing a product to satisfy every need of its potential user. The need exists first and the marketer will develop the product or service to satisfy the need as it exists. The seller, on the other hand, will concentrate on convincing the customer to accept the product as it exists.[3] In the beginning, the service was sold, not marketed. It was sold based on the perspectives and attitudes of the staff. The prevailing attitude was that the exchange process began and ended with Biomedical Information Service, as the producers.

The products offered for sale were the products easiest to produce. The needs assessed were the needs of Biomedical Information Service, not those of the clients. A quality product alone was believed enough to insure success.

The transition from selling to marketing had its start when the staff of Biomedical Information Service began to survey the available marketing literature. What started with the reading of one article has expanded into the application of marketing theory in the daily operation of this service. The first article read was Theodore Levitt's classic, "Marketing Myopia," and the excerpt which follows crystallized the drawbacks implicit in remaining a "seller."

> The railroads did not stop growing because the need for passenger and freight transportation declined. That grew. The railroads are in trouble today not because the need was filled by others (cars, trucks, airplanes, even telephones), but because they assumed themselves to be in the railroad business rather than in the transportation business. The reason they defined their industry wrong was because they were railroad-oriented instead of transportation-oriented; they were product-oriented instead of customer-oriented.[2]

Levitt speaks of railroads, but there is much to be learned by applying the same principles in a library setting. Creative application of marketing theory by a willing staff precludes obsolescence by anticipating and incorporating change, whether that change is generated by customer need or by available technology. Biomedical Information Service is currently making the transition from selling to marketing.

PRODUCT

The marketing process requires constant, long-term attention to detail. Each phase of the operation must be examined and marketing principles applied. Initially, the products of this service were examined. Product is the first "P" in the famous four "P's" of marketing—price, place or distribution, and promotion being the remaining three.[3] These four "P's" compose the foundation upon which marketing theory is built. Product rightly holds the first position. The product offered must meet the needs of specifically targeted markets and be of consistent and high quality. Many of the products offered by Biomedical Information Service have undergone refinement in order to better meet the needs of the targeted markets. One such market is attorneys.

Attorneys, as a market segment, represent thirty-five percent of the service's current volume. This client group needs information quickly. In response to that need, the average turnaround time was improved. In the first year of business, eighty-two percent of the orders for photocopying and ninety percent of the orders for computer-assisted research were completed in under twenty-four hours. In the second year, these figures improved to ninety-one and ninety-five percent respectively. It was discovered, however, in further assessing the needs of this client group, that even this was often not fast enough to meet their informational needs.

Rush services were then added to both photocopy and computer-assisted research. Rush service insures that the order takes priority over all other work; in fact, rush orders have been completed in as little as ten minutes. While these product refinements were initiated to meet the demands of a particular client group, all of the other clients have benefited. The achieved turnaround time holds for all orders received and rush service is available to all clients.

In scrutinizing production, Biomedical Information Service searched for ways to make each product more effective. Attorneys, a well-defined target market, will again serve as the example. This client group frequently needs to determine what has been published by a particular author and to locate those published materials. This need is normally met by performing computer-assisted research. Attorneys often use the information retrieved in this manner to verify their choice of a "medical expert" or to provide background on the expert who is testifying for opposing counsel. Once this particular informational need was understood, Biomedical Information Service was able to widen the range of resources which were applied and to expand the results. The informational need of attorneys was not necessarily confined to bibliographic information on what had been authored by a particular individual.

It typically included a biographical requirement as well. The Bio-Medical Library has the resources to provide this biographical background. Currently, any client requesting an author search is queried regarding his or her need for accompanying biographical information.

Surveying client requirements resulted in another product area which needed study: ease-of-use. Is it easy to access Biomedical Information Service? The answers given by clients to this question resulted in several changes. All phases of the operation were examined for ease-of-use. Initially, order placement by phone had been discouraged. Phone calls took time and interrupted work flow. Written orders, either sent in or dropped off took less processing time and allowed for better planning.

It was soon learned, however, that phone calls were the most convenient method of order placement for the majority of the clients. Two factors were involved. The first factor was time—theirs. They needed many of their orders handled immediately and did not choose to deal with the delays built into the existing system. It took less time for a client to call in an order than to compile a list and mail it to Biomedical Information Service. If the client called in, their order entered the work flow immediately. The second factor was personal contact. All clients like to feel their order will receive special attention. The contact afforded by the phone served to reassure the clients that their orders would be handled well and promptly. It also allowed them to ask questions regarding their order. Was billing possible? Could an order for photocopying be filled with incomplete citation information? How soon could their order be completed, and so on. They wanted their concerns answered, and in most cases, the mails did not meet their needs. Clients now are offered the option of phoning in, whether to place an order or to ask a question, and encouraged to use this option if it is the one they find most convenient.

As the ease-of-use issue continued to be examined, it became necessary to evaluate not only the convenience of access, but whether or not the resultant products were equally easy to use. Clients informed Biomedical Information Service that modifications were in order. Orders for photocopies were evaluated first. What did the client need with each photocopied article? This does fluctuate from one client to another, but there was a common denominator. All clients needed to know the source of the photocopied article. Therefore, all articles photocopied now have a copy of the client's citation, including the title of the journal, the volume and issue number, the date and the pages copied, attached to the first page of the article.

Next, the orders for computer-assisted research were assessed. Once clients had the results of the search, did they know how to read it and what to do with it? The answer, in many cases, was no. To correct this situation, three changes were instituted. The first involved the intake interview. The previous method of taking a search was augmented to include a broader explanation of the search results. The method of converting to a photocopy of the reference cited was explained. The availability of abstracts was also thoroughly explained and clients were encouraged to include this option when requesting a search. Secondly, an instructional sheet was developed which explained the meaning of each line on the computer printout. This sheet was included with every completed search. Thirdly, an individualized memo was sent with each search which discussed the results of that search and any available options for expanding the topic to yield additional information. These methods worked. Orders for computer-assisted research were increased by ninety-one percent in the second year of operation. Products continue to be tested to determine whether they meet the demands imposed by clients. As clients' needs change, so must the products.

PRICE

Price is the second of the four "P's" of marketing. Price refers to the exchange value placed on a given product. This value is determined by the perceived worth of the product, the prices charged by competing organizations and the costs involved in creating the product. Since the product of Biomedical Information Service is information, and this is a difficult commodity on which to place an appropriate market value,[4] consideration had to be given to the possibility of undervaluing as well as overvaluing the product. For example, a manual reference option is offered through Biomedical Information Service. Market research completed with clients indicated that this service had been undervalued.

Attorneys will again serve as the sample market segment. This group often needs manual reference services. In the beginning, manual reference was priced at thirty dollars per hour. This figure had been determined by comparing the rates charged by those perceived to be in competition with Biomedical Information Service. The competitors ranged in price per hour from twenty-five dollars to forty dollars. What was not considered in setting the price was the perceived value the clients would attach to the thirty dollar per hour rate. In the Minneapolis/St. Paul area, attorneys' fees range from sixty dollars per hour to one hundred and twenty dollars per hour. Paralegal time is billed out at thirty dollars per hour. At thirty dollars per hour, the rates for manual reference were the same as those of a paraprofessional in the legal field. It followed that lawyers would then perceive the manual reference option as being comparable to the work generated by a paraprofessional in their field. Since manual reference service is professional in nature, a compromise in exchange value was necessitated. Therefore the rate for manual reference was raised to forty dollars per hour.

If legal professionals bill out at a minimum of sixty dollars per hour, why was this not chosen as the exchange value? Attorneys, like all others engaged in private enterprise, must make a profit to survive. The sixty dollar per hour minimum is the rate charged to their client. Manual reference services had to be priced low enough to allow for a profit to the attorney, yet high enough to accurately express the value of services provided. The increase in price was applied to all clients. The decrease in usage which normally follows a price increase did not take place. Manual reference continues to be a growth area for this service.

Pricing was addressed again in the area of computer-assisted research. Many of the brokers who offer computer-assisted research charge for these services based on actual time, both online and staff time, spent in completing the search. While this is the easiest way for the producer to insure that the price charged covers the costs incurred, this method did not meet the clients' needs. Clients needed to know the cost of a search before it was run. Initially, searches were priced based on the average costs, for both online and personnel charges, collected over a one-year period. Seventy percent of the searches are performed on MEDLINE. For that reason, the price structure was initially attached to blocks of years, the search structure which already existed in that database. This method did not work. Money was lost on extensive searches requiring offline printouts and short, simple searches were overcharged. The clients were thoroughly confused by this pricing structure.

As a result a different cost configuration for computer-assisted research was recently developed. Prices for computer-assisted research are now based on the number of citations a client requires and the database used. The one thing that all clients had in common regarding database searching was that they always knew the quantity of citations they needed. They knew if their current project required ten citations, fifty citations, one hundred or one thousand, and a price structure which reflected this quantification resulted in ready understanding.

Price was also of prime consideration as the placement of orders by phone began to be encouraged. As previously stated, taking phone orders interrupted work flow and giving appropriate service to each phone customer put a large burden on a small staff. A compromise became imperative as the volume of requests increased. Initially, phone orders were penalized by considering an order received in this manner a rush order, therefore, an additional five dollars per citation was charged. This position was reviewed by applying marketing techniques, and the error was realized, yet a way was needed to mediate the difference between the clients' convenience and the shortage of Biomedical Information Service staff. A balance was struck between these two needs.

Two separate price structures evolved for photocopy service. Any order placed by phone was to be charged at a rate of five dollars per article plus ten cents per page. Any order placed with this service in printed form receives a sixty percent discount off the aforementioned price, and is filled for two dollars per article plus ten cents per page. The higher price for phone orders helped offset the personnel costs incurred in handling those orders. This method solved the problem while allowing clients to choose the service level their order required. Orders phoned in receive individualized attention at the time of placement, and immediately enter the work flow. Orders placed in printed form receive comparable attention upon receipt, but do not involve staff time in placing the order.

This pricing method is mutually beneficial. It allows clients to prioritize their order in terms of attention and urgency while also allowing them the advantage of a price break on orders not requiring immediate attention. Simultaneously, it allows Biomedical Information Service staff to focus attention on those clients and orders that most require it. The number of orders placed in each pricing option continues to grow annually, indicating that this price split is an effective reconciliation.

PLACE

Place or distribution is the third marketing "P" to be considered. At this time, the "place" of operation is established. We are physically located within the University of Minnesota. The Bio-Medical Library's financial picture will not currently allow the establishment of outposts for the service, although this concept has been considered. Place can also refer to the geographic area served. Biomedical Information Service, being a part of a tax supported, land-grant academic institution, has a responsibility to those people who help to support the institution. For that reason, clients within the state of Minnesota are the primary focus, although no client is refused service on the basis of location. Further discussion of the third marketing "P," place, will center on the related concept of distribution.

Currently, the products of this service are distributed in many ways, depending solely upon the client's sense of urgency, and on their location. In the beginning, however, only three distribution possibilities were offered. Clients could pick up their orders; they could have their order sent out by U.S. Mail; or, if they had a University of Minnesota mailing address, they could take advantage of the free intracampus mailing system. For many clients, none of these options met their needs. After applying marketing methodology to this problem, customized delivery was initiated. All possible methods now are utilized in order to deliver the product within the time constraints imposed by clients. Accounts have been established by Biomedical Information Service with various courier services, cab companies, express mail services, airlines and electronic mail services. The method which best meets the client's criterion is the method employed.

Perhaps the best way to illustrate the lengths to which Biomedical Information Service will go to meet clients' needs in the area of distribution is to cite an actual case. A phone call was received at ten o'clock one Wednesday morning from a client located in Montana. The client needed photocopies of six articles to be completed by two o'clock that same afternoon; these articles were to be delivered to the Minneapolis Airport where they would be picked up by a passenger changing flights, on his way to Duluth, with a twenty minute layover. This client needed the information for a presentation which he was to give on his arrival in Duluth. The photocopies were completed, the passenger service manager of the airline involved was contacted, and the packet was delivered to the manager, who, in turn, passed it on to the manager of the next work shift, who delivered it to the client as he ran to make his flight connection! All in a day's marketing. While this type of customized delivery does not occur daily, Biomedical Information Service is ready when the need arises.

PROMOTION

Promotion is the final marketing concept which was considered. This concept is the one which comes most readily to mind when the subject of marketing surfaces, but it is rightfully the last in terms of priority. Promotion comes after product, price and place have been addressed.[3] The promotional methods used by Biomedical Information Service are many and varied, but the first concern remains word-of-mouth advertising. This has been called both the worst and best method of advertising, and rightly so. A satisfied client will tell colleagues about the existence of a service when, and if, the appropriate time and circumstance arises. A dissatisfied client will expound in loud terms, to anyone who will listen upon the wrongful treatment received. Biomedical Information Service will do almost anything necessary to prove the service subscribes to the theory that the "customer is always right." Biomedical Information Service strives to have its word-of-mouth promotion be only positive.

While word-of-mouth advertising is certainly effective, its exclusive usage results in slow growth rates. Therefore, Biomedical Information Service has supplemented this promotional method with a number of other efforts. Direct mail marketing has proven to be a cost-effective promotional tool for this service. Biomedical Information Service has developed and maintains its own mailing list, which is housed in a mini-computer owned by the library. The mailing list currently contains over seven thousand names. The direct mail pieces produced are aimed at specific target markets, with each market's needs being individually addressed in the manner in which the promotional piece is written and designed. The format most often used to court a target market is a postcard. Postcards are inexpensive to produce and may enjoy a lower bulk mail rate than a larger piece. The one thing every postcard produced has in common is a call-to-action.

Ordinarily, the call-to-action is an invitation to call or write for more extensive information on the services available. The more the prospective client becomes involved, the more likely that person is to use the service. A call-to-action is imperative. The "more extensive information" is sent to potential clients who respond to the postcard and takes the form of a generic brochure, appropriate to all clients, and a personalized, signed letter inviting the prospective client to call for a free consultation to discuss their informational needs. In addressing smaller, or new target markets, individualized word-processor letters are oftentimes appropriate and allow the testing of different promotional approaches.

Although direct mail marketing is a cost-effective method, it too can be supplemented. The public relations department of the University of Minnesota has helped immensely with the promotional efforts. This department has prepared press releases about Biomedical Information Service and also has produced articles which have appeared in various Univesity publications. They have provided Biomedical Information Service with copies of each of their efforts which have then been incorporated into the promotional programs established by this service.

Biomedical Information Service also has prepared its own news releases and sent them to area newsletters. Since many of these publications are continually seeking information to pass on to their readers, this method has worked well. Biomedical Information Service staff members are about to begin an ongoing informational column for one such newsletter, which will serve well from the standpoint of name recognition, a high priority in all of the promotional work. Although each of these methods has its own merit, all promotional efforts are useless without satisfied customers. Ultimately, the most energetic effort in promotional terms is exerted in maintaining relationships with established clients and to make certain the needs of those clients are well satisfied.

Marketing efforts are ongoing. The search continues for ways to make this service more responsive to the needs of its clients. Attitudes have changed. Methods have improved. Volume has increased consistently. The needs of Biomedical Information Service no longer come first. The informational needs the clients are willing to entrust to this service have also expanded. The days of "selling" are gone. Marketing has had a vital impact, and new applications for it are found in the ongoing effort to increase the viability of this service.

REFERENCES

1. Baker, Michael J., ed. *Marketing in Adversity*. New York: Macmillan Press, LTD, 1976.

2. Levitt, Theodore. "Marketing Myopia." *Harvard Business Review* 53 (1975): 26ff.

3. Lunden, Elizabeth. "Marketing and the R.I.C.E. Operation." In *Conference on Fee-based Research in College and University Libraries*. Proceedings of the meetings at C. W. Post Center of Long Island University. Greenvale, New York. June 17–18, 1982. New York: C. W. Post Center of Long Island University, 1982, pp. 114.

4. Oldman, Christine. "Marketing Library and Information Services." *European Journal of Marketing* 11 (1977):460–74.

SELECTED BIBLIOGRAPHY

Boss, Richard W. "The Library as an Information Broker." *College and Research Libraries* 40 (March 1979):136–40.

Freeman, James E., and Katz, Ruth M. "Information Marketing." In: *Annual Re-*

view of Information Science and Technology, v. 13, edited by Martha Williams. New York: Knowledge Industry Publications, 1978, pp. 37–59.

Jackson, A. R. Haygarth. "Publicity or Selling the Information Service." *ASLIB Proceedings* 25 (October 1973):385–9.

Kotler, Philip. "Strategies for Introducing Marketing into Nonprofit Organizations." *Journal of Marketing* 43 (January 1979):37–44.

Kotler, Philip. "Strategic Planning and the Marketing Process." *Business* 30 (May–June 1980):2–9.

Kotler, Philip. *Marketing for Nonprofit Organizations.* 2d ed. New Jersey: Prentice-Hall, Inc., 1982.

Lunden, Elizabeth. "The Library as a Business." *American Libraries* 13 (July 1982):471–2.

Maranjian, Lorig, and Boss, Richard W. *Fee-based Information Services: A Study of a Growing Industry.* London: R. R. Bowker, 1980.

Shapiro, Benson P. "Marketing for Nonprofit Organizations." *Harvard Business Review* 51 (September–October 1973):123–32.

Shapiro, Stanley J. "Marketing and the Information Professional: Odd Couple or Meaningful Relationship?" *Special Libraries* 71 (November 1980): 469–74.

Thompson, James C. "Regional Information and Communication Exchange: A Case Study." In: *Conference on Fee-based Research in College and University Libraries.* Proceedings of the meetings at C. W. Post Center of Long Island University. Greenvale, New York. June 17–18, 1982. New York: C. W. Post Center of Long Island University, 1982, pp. 55–76.

Urquhart, D. J. "Economic Analysis of Information Services." *Journal of Documentation* 32 (June 1976):123–5.

Weinstock, M. "Marketing Scientific and Technical Information Service." In: *Encyclopedia of Library and Information Science* v. 17, edited by Allen Kent. New York: Marcel Dekker, 1976, pp. 165–88.

Wood, Elizabeth. "Strategic Planning and the Marketing Process: Library Applications." *Journal of Academic Librarianship* 9 (March 1983): 15–20.

IV. FEE-FOR-SERVICE

The "free or fee" issue has been a major subject of debate. With the increasing emphasis on cost recovery, fees for library services have become commonplace in health sciences libraries. Specialized services such as online search services are routinely offered for a fee in most libraries. Foreman, in her overview of fee-for-service in publicly funded libraries, views fee-for-service programs as a means of ensuring access to information. A long-standing, well-established fee-for-service system, involving library membership and service fees, is described by Hill. Beecher, on the other hand, discusses the implementation of a new fee-based information service and the role of libraries in offering services to non-primary clientele. As a contrast to library-based information services, Stefanacci and Martin describe the founding and management of an information brokerage.

Fee-for-Service
in Publicly Supported Libraries:
An Overview

Gertrude E. Foreman

ABSTRACT. The principle of open access to information is shared by most librarians. The fee-for-service concept has been regarded as contradictory; however, fee-for-service programs for nonprimary clientele can play an important role in ensuring access to information.

INTRODUCTION

The principle of open and equitable access to information is shared by most librarians in publicly supported academic institutions, including access to collections and services by clients who are not affiliated with the libraries' parent institutions. To many, access to information is regarded as a prerogative of all Americans because, proponents contend, an informed citizenry is for the public good. These long held beliefs are being challenged in recent years as an increasing number of libraries have initiated user fees to support or subsidize services, especially those based on new technology. Fees for service is not a new concept for libraries, but the demand for service by various client groups, with the accompanying higher costs, has resulted in self supporting service programs which academic librarians find acceptable. An exploration of the trends, issues, philosophy, and program plans for user charges suggests that fee-for-service has a legitimate role in publicly funded academic libraries.

Gertrude E. Foreman is Head of Reference Services at the Bio-Medical Library, University of Minnesota, Minneapolis, MN. She received her M. L. S. from the University of Minnesota Library School. As a long time searcher, she has been involved in fees for database search services since 1974.

OVERVIEW OF USER FEE ISSUES

The charging of user fees by publicly funded libraries is not a new phenomenon. Many public and academic libraries in the United States were charging user fees by the late 1800s.[1] Over the years, fees have been charged for interlibrary loans, bibliographic compilations, special equipment and materials, meeting rooms, special reference services, and photocopying.

That fees are quite widely accepted in academic libraries is obvious from a survey conducted by the Systems and Procedures Exchange Center of the Association of Research Libraries in 1980.[2] The survey revealed that all sixty responding libraries charged for photoduplication and most charged for online searching. In a survey of public and academic libraries, Blazek reported that "attitude toward user fees is a function of the type of library in which employed" and concluded that "public reference librarians were more opposed to user fees than were academic reference librarians at any level."[3]

During the last two decades, academic libraries have changed from passive institutions, with a primary goal of collection building, to active institutions which provide a wide range of special information services determined by user needs. Most of these expanded services were based on new technologies, including computers and media, or were oriented toward the needs of individuals or small groups, such as online database services, selective dissemination of information, or bibliographic instruction. Without adequate financial support for all the services, libraries initiated user charges. Areas of special interest have been online database searching and external user services.

Few issues in librarianship during the past ten years have resulted in so much controversy as that of user charges, especially for one of the new services—online database search services. With the introduction of online searching, librarians faced a problem of providing an innovative but expensive service. Furthermore, online searching was characterized as (1) a highly customized product; (2) a transaction of significant and identifiable cost; and (3) a labor-intensive service requiring considerable librarian time and responsibility.[4] Defined in these terms, it was less difficult to make the decision to charge a fee for online services. Then, too, printed index counterparts were available for many databases, thus online searching could be regarded as an additional, alternative service. The librarians' debate over user fees tended to obscure the more important issue of the changing roles of libraries and librarians.

The debate over database search charges did help clarify issues regarding fee for services. Some individuals argue that user fees will have a negative impact on access to information.[5] Others see the user fees as beneficial to libraries by making possible new and expanded services.[6] Librarians opposed to charges argue that user fees: (1) impede access to information which is necessary in a democratic society; (2) discriminate against users who lack the money to pay; (3) represent a double taxation in publicly supported libraries; (4) may result in a reduction of public support through taxes; and (5) will encourage libraries to place greater emphasis on fee-based services. Proponents of fee-based service content that user fees (1) provide the library with funds to expand its user services; (2) provide planning information; (3) minimize excessive utilization of services; and (4) provide a method for determining use of limited library resources.[7]

Like online database searching, services for external or nonprimary clientele have come under scrutiny, especially during periods of declining budgets. Librarians have begun to question whether services traditionally offered to nonprimary clientele conflict with their ability to serve primary clients. At the same time, the demand for information by the public is increasing. Generally, this reflects the "knowledge economy,"[8] while medical librarians, specifically, might point to the consumer health movement, continuing education requirements, growth in biotechnology, and changing roles of health professionals. In publicly supported libraries, it is difficult to deny access to information by taxpaying clients with such valid and critical information needs. Some libraries have controlled use by establishing use policies and/or imposing user fees.

External user policies are common in academic libraries. These usually consist of statements on general access, borrowing, and reference services and on differential pricing for bibliographic searching or photocopy services. In a survey of the Association of Research Libraries' members, sixty-one of sixty-four institutions surveyed had written formal policies for external user services and nineteen had instituted user fees.[9] These policies often address the academic library's commitment to external users. One tax-supported, land-grant institution's policy states that the "best interests of the community and state are served when our resources are available to industry, research, and business," and concludes that "while we recognize the obligations to respond to the needs arising from non-academic sources, the primary professional responsibility of the librarian is to the University. No service should be undertaken that might interfere with the discharge of this duty."[10]

There is considerable variation in the fee structure for services in academic libraries. Most publicly supported libraries provide access to collections and on-site reference service to all clients. Where charges are imposed for a library service, such as photocopying or online bibliographic searching, the external user often pays an additional fee. Increasingly, libraries are establishing special departments or service units with the primary purpose of serving external users, especially corporate or business clients. These services are available at prices which are significantly higher than those charged for their primary user group.

In their study of pricing of online services for nonprimary clients, Beeler and Lueck provide a convincing rationale for a price discrimination policy for nonprofit organizations. Price discrimination is defined as the "practice of charging various prices to different customers for the same product."[11] Although publicly supported libraries do not have a profit motive, price discrimination serves other goals. First, it does generate income to cover costs. Second, it can reduce demand for a service, such as online searches, by nonprimary clientele, thus allowing searchers more time to provide service to primary clients. And, third, the concept of just pricing is applicable to libraries. An example of just pricing is that primary clients are charged a "flat fee" or a subsidized fee because they have made prior payment through tuition. Beeler and Lueck conclude that "it is appropriate, and often desirable, for prices to reflect considerations other than cost."[12]

RETHINKING USER FEE ISSUES

In examining the current state of user fees in publicly supported libraries, it is apparent that academic libraries have accepted the idea more readily than have public libraries. In academic libraries, fees are often charged for photocopying and online bibliographic searching. Furthermore, these academic libraries often charge nonprimary users a higher fee for services. Much of the debate regarding user fees has centered on fees for primary clientele; but for many librarians, the concept of charging for services in publicly supported libraries is unacceptable. Even when budget constraints required that charges be imposed if the service was to be offered, the fee structure may be established with misgivings.

Like all professionals, librarians share certain assumptions, values, and beliefs which are reflected not only in practice but in codes and policies as well. The American Library Association (ALA) statement on Professional Ethics calls for "freedom of access to information" and a "special obligation to ensure the free flow of information and ideas to present and future generations."[13] The ALA policy manual has as a number one policy to "promote efforts to assure every individual access to needed information."[14] In its Positions and Public Policy Statement section, ALA supports "Goals for Action" of the National Commission on Libraries and Information Science (NCLIS). Under the title, "Free Access to Information," the policy states that "the American Library Association asserts that the charging of fees and levies for information services, including those services utilizing the latest information technology, is discriminatory in publicly supported institutions providing library and information services."[15] According to an NCLIS report, one role for the library is to provide "equity in access" to information.[16] Thus, many librarians have accepted free and equitable access as a basic value and this value has been translated into a policy.

The decision to provide service for fees takes place in a single library, by individuals, for a certain clientele. "It is only natural," Blazek writes, "for librarians to entertain doubts about the wisdom of their decisions. . . ."[17] Feelings of anxiety and dissonance accompany decisions which run counter to commonly held values. The librarian may counter this feeling by seeking a rationale that makes charging fees acceptable. This often takes the form of reasons that refute the anti-fee sentiments.[18] Another approach is to reevaluate our values and beliefs related to information access.

Is free and equitable access to information still a valid ethical tenet? Most librarians would answer "yes," while recognizing that, in the application of the tenet, there is considerable variation. For example, people recognize that, although all have freedom of speech, some broadcast their views from a soapbox while others have access to national television; but this difference does not negate the right to freedom of speech. Other professions have struggled with similar dilemmas concerning equity. A notable example is the right to equality in health care. Charles Fried argues that "the real task. . .is not. . .to explain why there must be complete equality in medicine, but the more subtle and perilous task of determining the decent minimum in respect to health which accords with sound ethical judgments, while maintaining the virtues of freedom, variety, and flexibility. . . ."[19]

Although the concept of a decent minimum might seem harsh at first glance, it is, in fact, an ethical view. Many librarians use the concept in establishing reference policies, especially in times of limited staffing. When a librarian provides a five minute database search free, but refers the client to their fee-based service for more comprehensive searching, the librarian is providing a decent minimum of access. Or when the librarian allocates ten minutes for a telephone reference question from a nonprimary client, the decent minimum concept has been used.

Librarians who must set levels for decent minimum service will welcome fee-for-service programs as a referral point for clients requesting more extensive services. The establishment of fee-based services for external use can provide access without deleterious effects on service to primary clientele. To the contrary, the well managed fee-based service can enhance the library by providing income, additional staff, and a positive image to the public. Upon observing these advantages, an increasing number of libraries are establishing fee-based service programs.

FEE-BASED SERVICE PROGRAMS

Fee-based services have found an accepted place in publicly supported academic libraries. Piternick, in an excellent case history of fee for services, writes that the "library of a publicly supported institution cannot provide unlimited services to the public. . .at the cost of jeopardizing services to its primary users. . . ."[20] A number of successful fee-based service programs suggests that other librarians share Piternick's view. At the University of Minnesota, the Bio-Medical Library, St. Paul Campus Library, and the Engineering Library have initiated services for external users after careful planning to make certain primary user services are enhanced, not diminished.[21] Although not documented, Bio-Medical Library staff sense that their Biomedical Information Service (BIS) has helped alleviate some reference desk work loads, both telephone and on site, by serving corporate clients. The Georgia Institute of Technology has had a successful information program for many years.[22] Long Island University's Center for Business Research serves students as well as corporate firms.[23] The Regional Information and Communication Exchange (R.I.C.E.) at Rice University, a private not publicly supported institution, is a well-known model for other libraries.[24,25] Richards and Cody report on a new service at Lehigh University for the business and industrial community.[26] The University of Pittsburgh provides service to business and industry through the NASA Industrial Applications Center (NIAS). At the University of Colorado, the Colorado Technical Reference Center's (CTRC) fact sheets and newsletter list a wide variety of services for external clientele. Michigan Information Transfer Service (MITS), provides similar services at the University of Michigan, as does the Information Services Division of the Kurt F. Wendt Library at the University of Wisconsin. Although some programs are separate administration units, these fee-for-service models are applicable to the academic library.

CONCLUSION

The principle of free and equitable access to information is a basic tenet of librarianship. Fee-for-service programs have been regarded with considerable hostility in the past, but this attitude is moderating as librarians attempt to provide service to both their primary clientele and to an ever increasing number of external users. Fee-for-service programs can play an important role in ensuring that all clients, in fact, do have access to needed information.

REFERENCES

1. Waldhart, T.J., and Bellardo, T. "User Fees in Publicly Funded Libraries." In: *Advances in Librarianship*. Vol. 9, Harris, M.H., ed. New York: Academic Press, 1979, pp. 31–61.

2. Association of Research Libraries. Office of Management Studies. *Fees For Services*. Washington, D.C.: Association of Research Libraries, 1981. Systems and Procedure Exchange Center, SPEC KIT #74.

3. Blazek, R. "User Fees: A Survey of Public and Academic Reference Librarians." *Reference Librarian* 4 (Summer 1982):55–74.

4. DeWath, N.V. "Fees for Online Bibliographic Search Services in Publicly Supported Libraries." *Library Research* 3 (Spring 1981):29–45.

5. Blake, F.M., and Perlmutter, E.L. "The Rush to User Fees: Alternative Proposals." *Library Journal* 102 (October 1, 1977):2005–8.

6. DeGennaro, R. "Pay Libraries and User Charges." *Library Journal* 100 (February 15, 1975):363–7.

7. Waldhart and Bellardo, p. 47.

8. Drucker, Peter. *The Age of Discontinuity*. New York: Harper & Row, 1969.

9. Association of Research Libraries. Office of Management Studies. *External User Services*. Washington, D.C.: Association of Research Libraries, 1981. Systems and Procedure Exchange Center, SPEC KIT #73.

10. Ibid., p. 61.

11. Beeler, R.J., and Lueck, A.L. "Pricing of Online Services for Nonprimary Clientele." *Journal of Academic Librarianship* 10 (May 1984):67–72.

12. Ibid., p. 72.

13. "ALA Statement on Professional Ethics." *American Libraries* 12 (June 1981):335.

14. American Library Association. *Handbook of Organization, 1981–82*. ALA Policy Manual, Sec. 1, p. 176. Chicago: ALA, 1981.

15. Ibid., p. 185.

16. United States. National Commission on Libraries and Information Science. Public Section/Private Sector Task Force. *Public Sector/Private Sector Interaction in Providing Information Services*. Washington, D.C.: GPO, 1982.

17. Ibid., p. 33.

18. Freeman, J.E., and Katz, R. M. "Information Marketing." *Annual Review of Information Science and Technology* 13 (1978):79–101.

19. Fried, C. "Equality and Rights in Medical Care." *Hastings Center Rep.* 6 (February 1976):29–34.

20. Piternick, A. B. "Problems of Resource Sharing With the Community." *Journal of Academic Librarianship* 5 (July 1979):153–8.

21. O'Connell, K., and Freeman, J. K. "The Development of a Fee-Based Service in an Academic Health Science Library." Paper presented at the 84th Annual Meeting, Medical Library Association, May 25–31, 1984, Denver, Colorado.

22. Dodd, J.B. "Ins and Outs of Charging for Research Services." In: *Confer-*

ence on *Fee-Based Research in College and University Libraries.* Proceedings of the meetings at C.W. Post Center of Long Island University, Greenvale, N.Y., June 17–18, 1982, pp. 20–34.

23. Grant, M.M. "The Center for Business Research: A Case Study." In: *Conference on Fee-Based Research in College and University Libraries,* pp. 77–85.

24. Thompson, J.C. Regional Information and Community Exchange: A Case Study." In: *Conference on Fee-Based Research in College and University Libraries,* pp. 55–76.

25. Lunden, E. "Marketing and the R.I.C.E. Operation." In: *Conference on Fee-Based Research in College and University Libraries,* pp. 113–27.

26. Richards, B.G., and Cody, S.A. "A New Fee-Based Information Service in an Academic Library." In: *Conference on Fee-Based Research in College and University Libraries,* pp. 128–32.

Example of a Complex Fee-for-Service System

Susan Hill

ABSTRACT. The fee-for-service component of the Cleveland Health Sciences Library (CHSL) is described, giving the history of the system and showing the evolution and growth of a library which provides a variety of services to a university, to area health practitioners, and to institutions in Northeastern Ohio. Approximately 15 percent of the total budget has been recovered annually from membership and service fees during the fifteen years CHSL has served a private medical society, an institutional membership, and a university population.

Descriptions of fee-for-service programs in particular libraries help to illustrate the ways libraries have adapted to the surrounding community, to the demands of users, and to the various philosophies of mission held by their administrators, managers, boards, and faculties. The Cleveland Health Sciences Library (CHSL) serves as an interesting example of a complex system of services and programs, some of which have evolved into models for efforts in other libraries.

The CHSL librarians have grappled with the problems of balance among its various programs and memberships and also have evaluated the library's national, regional and local networks in terms of providing effective user services. Fees for services provided beyond the Case Western Reserve University population have been systematized into programs which also can serve as useful models of ways to enhance a library's budgetary base.

Susan Hill is Interlibrary Loan Librarian at Cleveland Health Sciences Library (CHSL). She received an M.S.L.S. and an M.A. in English from Case Western Reserve University. She has served as Assistant Reference and Audiovisual Librarian, and for almost eight years as a Catalog Librarian prior to taking over Interlibrary Loan in 1981.

HISTORICAL PERSPECTIVE

Cleveland Health Sciences Library has operated throughout its history on a fee-for-service basis. Organized library access originated for Cleveland health care professionals with the Cleveland Medical Library Association (CMLA) in 1894. Formation of that organization culminated efforts of three early medical societies to create a library through mutual participation and contributions. Annual dues were pledged at $10 during the year 1895, and afforded members of the CMLA access to about 2,000 donated and purchased volumes. Both books and periodicals were gathered including some gifts of rare and prized items. The location changed from Case Library downtown in Cleveland to an old residence at 586 Prospect Street, and finally after the Association gained substantial funds, it erected a magnificent building in 1925.[1] The library was dedicated the Dudley P. Allen Memorial Library November 13, 1926. The building is now a National Historic Landmark.

The Cleveland Medical Library Association continues as a strong personal membership supporting the Cleveland Health Sciences Library, which was formed July 1, 1966 when proposals for collaboration between CMLA and Case Western Reserve University came to fruition. The Health Center Library building was completed in 1971 and consolidated the previously separate collections of the CWRU schools of Dentistry, Medicine, Nursing and the departments of Nutrition and Biology. Now Case Western Reserve University health sciences students have additional areas of interest such as biomedical engineering, biometry, and medical anthropology which are supported by the Library's collections. Materials are divided between the two libraries as follows: users of the Health Center Library are generally involved in education in pure sciences, preclinical training and research; users of the Allen Library are usually clinicians. There is a free flow of users daily between the two nearby facilities which make up the Cleveland Health Sciences Library.

In 1968/69 the Library initiated an institutional membership which afforded services to area hospitals. Reference, online access, interlibrary loan, photocopy, and consultation were offered on a cost recovery basis.[2] From an initial membership of twelve hospital libraries in 1969, institutional membership has grown to over 180 in 1984. Institutions now include law firms, educational and commercial health care organizations, chemical companies, and many hospitals. From a membership/endowment supported library from 1894 through 1966, to the complex organization serving a diverse clientele in 1984, the Cleveland Health Sciences Library has continued to recover part of its budget from dues and service fees.

IMPACT OF THE REGIONAL MEDICAL LIBRARY NETWORK

Since the early seventies the Cleveland Health Sciences Library, along with most major medical libraries, has experienced dramatic growth in its user population and the demand for services. As a Resource Library in the National Library of Medicine's Regional Medical Library Network, CHSL also experienced an accelerated growth of institutional membership, in part due to the structured aspect of the network and also because of document delivery referral guidelines. Requests for document delivery were passed from "basic units" to the Resource Libraries, into the broader regional network, and lastly on to the National Library of Medicine (NLM). Unparalleled expansion in document delivery caused CHSL to become one of the largest lenders in the United States with over 45,000 filled requests in 1982/83. From 75 percent to 80 percent of the document delivery activity was for personal CMLA members in area hospitals and for institutional members of the Library, as well as other institutions in the CHSL service area.

Document delivery services outside of the service area were reimbursed by the NLM, but only about one percent to two percent of the total library budget was recovered from federal reimbursement to CHSL. When price support for document delivery ended January 1, 1981, Cleveland Health Sciences Library continued to participate as a Resource Library. Due to the previous fee-for-service arrangement with CHSL, area institutions did not experience a difference in fees at the end of federal reimbursement and only had to cope with new charges and increases in fees from other Resource Libraries and from NLM. Since the NLM regions were reconfigured in 1983, CHSL has remained the largest lender in the new Region 3. Cleveland Health Sciences Library handled approximately 30 percent of the total document delivery traffic throughout the duration of the previous Kentucky-Ohio-Michigan Regional Medical Library Program.

IMPACT OF OTHER NETWORK ACTIVITIES

The CHSL also participates in two other local networks which have provided enhanced ability to serve its users. The Northeastern Ohio Major Academic Libraries (NEOMAL) cooperate to provide interlibrary loan requests at unusual speed among nine large colleges and universities. The Cleveland Area Metropolitan Library System (CAMLS) serves to involve the CHSL with community libraries of many types, and provides another avenue for obtaining material on interlibrary loan. Both networks have enhanced a variety of services the Library has been able to provide its personal and institutional members, and a review of costs involved in participation in each of the major networks has shown that benefits have equaled the expense of participation.

POPULATIONS SERVED AND PERCENTAGES OF BUDGET RECOVERED

In 1984 the Library served approximately 5,000 faculty, staff, and health sciences students at Case Western Reserve University, 1,700 personal members of the Cleveland Medical Library Association, and 180 institutional members. Budgetary support by group is as follows: 69 percent of the total budget is provided by Case Western Reserve University schools; 15 percent of the total budget derives from the membership dues for personal and institutional members, the circuit program, and service fees, and 16 percent of the total budget is generated from endowment and other sources. The total budget was approximately two million dollars in 1983/84.

PERSONAL LIBRARY MEMBERSHIP

Personal membership in the Cleveland Medical Library Association is available in three basic categories: "Members" are individuals who wish to use the collections and services of the Library; "Fellows" pay an increased fee annually and a one time fee of $100, and are eligible for membership on CMLA Committees and election to the Board of Trustees; and "Fellows for Life" pay a one time fee of $1,000, and are exempt from dues for life. They also receive free photocopy and online services. The Library also has categories of "Junior Member" which allows teaching hospital house staff to use the collections, and for "Honorary" and "Emeritus" members. The overall rationale behind personal CMLA membership has been to assess dues for general library support and to provide access to library services for individuals who are doing personal research. The library in an institution in which a personal member is active is conceived as the primary resource for information needs pertaining to his or her work in that institution. Personal membership in the Cleveland Medical Library Association in addition implies a special desire to support the Association's activities and to utilize the collections and services of the Cleveland Health Sciences Library. The benefits of personal membership include online access, reference services, interlibrary loan, photocopy service at a moderate fee, and general access to the facilities and collections. Figure 1 is a chart of personal member categories and services.

INSTITUTIONAL MEMBERSHIP

The strategy for charging institutional members, on the other hand, has evolved quite a bit over its relatively short (fifteen year) history. The method for charging has changed more often because of the continuing effort to achieve a fair division of support among area institutions using CHSL. In addition, an attempt has been made to achieve balanced support between institutions with many CMLA members and institutions with no CMLA members. Both fixed and variable fees were tried, and finally as in the case of personal member-

FIGURE 1

PERSONAL MEMBERSHIP CATEGORIES/SERVICES

	DUES	ONLINE SEARCH	QUICK REFERENCE	CITATION VERIFICATION	LOAN OF MATERIAL	PHOTOCOPY SERVICE	INTERLIBRARY LOAN
NON MEMBER	---	$20 Medline; Others depend on cost	FREE	Not Available	$6 per Item	$6 per Item	$6 per Item
HOUSE STAFF	$5	Not Available	FREE	Not Available	FREE	Not Available	Not Available
CWRU FACULTY	---	FREE	FREE	25 free; 50¢ per Citation	FREE	$2 per Item	FREE
CWRU STUDENTS	---	FREE	FREE	Not Available	FREE	Not Available	FREE
CMLA MEMBERS	$35	FREE	FREE	25 FREE; 50¢ per Citation	FREE	$2 per Item	FREE
CMLA FELLOWS	$100 once; $50/yr.	FREE	FREE	25 FREE; 50¢ per Citation	FREE	$2 per Item	FREE
CMLA EMERITUS & HONORARY MEMBERS	---	FREE	FREE	25 FREE; 50¢ per Citation	FREE	$2 per Item	FREE
CMLA FELLOWS FOR LIFE	$1,000 Once	FREE	FREE	25 FREE; 50¢ per Citation	FREE	FREE	FREE

ship, a combination was chosen. In 1972 institutions paid a single fixed fee which was set according to a complex formula based on size and relative use of services. Since 1977, a fixed fee has been set at a standard rate for all institutions with a unit charge for transactions for interlibrary loan/photocopy, online access, consultation, or in the case of circuit libraries for the additional expenses related to that service. The mixture of fixed and variable fees is easily applied and is most acceptable and understandable from the point of view of the institutions.

Institutional membership in the Cleveland Health Sciences Library contains three membership categories:

1. Category "A" institutional members are fully operational libraries with full-time professionals or library technicians. These libraries are expected to function quite independently in acquiring information and services not available at CHSL.
2. Category "B" members are law firms and other commercial health care organizations which do not have full-time librarians and for whom CHSL is the primary library. CHSL provides these institutions much enhanced reference service as well as expanded interlibrary loan service at an additional fee. The library allows individual users in the Type B institutions to use a simple in-house request form.
3. Type "C" institutions are circuit libraries operated through the circuit librarianship program. The circuit program recovers costs and has run independently since 1973. Cost recovery in the circuit program is described elsewhere in this monographic supplement.

The fixed fee of $100 per year pertains to all categories. Transaction fees vary slightly by category. A chart of institutional member categories and their dues and services appears as Figure 2.

Through differentiated service categories, institutional members receive tailored services in order to meet their particular needs effectively. Use of the Resource Library by Type A institutional members tends to follow an even pattern reflecting their well-developed in-house library services. Use of the library by Type B institutions tends to be low or sporadic, and to follow an extremely uneven pattern of demand. Especially the needs of the small law firms and commercial enterprises using the health sciences literature had not previously been met through conventional library access since these institutions did not have a full-time person devoted to serving as "librarian." The circuit institutions (Type C) generally show higher use of the Resource Library for their relative size due to the advantage of having circuit librarians who spend one day per week at CHSL attending to their needs.

FIGURE 2

INSTITUTIONAL DUES AND SERVICES

CATEGORIES	DUES	ONLINE SEARCH	QUICK REFERENCE	LOAN OF MATERIAL	PHOTOCOPY SERVICE	INTERLIBRARY LOAN	CONSULTATION
TYPE A (With Libraries)	$100	$10 Medline; Others depend on cost	FREE	$3 per Item	$3 per Item	$3 per Referral	$25 per hour
TYPE B (Without Libraries)	$100	$10 Medline; Others depend on cost	FREE	$3 per Item	$3 per Item	$3 per Item	$25 per hour
TYPE C (Circuits)	$100	$10 Medline; Others depend on cost	FREE	$2 per Item	$2 per Item	$2 per Item	$25 per hour
NON MEMBER	---	$20 Medline; Others depend on cost	FREE	$6 per Item	$6 per Item	Not Available	$25 per hour

The circuit institutions represent a group of institutions with needs which are met in a more formal program than that of the other categories.

Generally, growth of in-house services tends to increase external service demands. The more a service such as online searching is provided by an institution to its own users, the greater the demand for the service becomes; demand for external services such as interlibrary loan rises proportionally. Over time most institutional members have increased their use of the CHSL.

UNIVERSITY POPULATION

The Cleveland Health Sciences Library serves its diverse CWRU population without fees for service. A large percentage of the total library budget (60 percent) derives from the CWRU health sciences schools of Nursing, Medicine, Dentistry, and the departments of Nutrition and Biology. Only unusually expensive database searches or interlibrary loans are charged back to university patrons. Health sciences faculty of CWRU are considered to have the benefits of regular personal CMLA members. The house staff of area teaching hospitals have direct access to the CHSL collections as "Junior Members" of the CMLA, whose dues are often paid by the hospital.

DUES AND SERVICE FEES: GENERAL CONCEPTS

In 1975 the Cleveland Health Sciences Library was the site for a CWRU Department of Economics dissertation entitled "Library Pricing Models and Information Requirements: a Case Study" by Cheryl Casper.[3] Her study pointed out some important thoughts regarding library charges. User fees may be levied to generate revenue, to ration demand for given services, or to provide information about the value of the service (if, for example, demand falls/rises when a price is levied) as a management tool. A library's objective in setting user fees is not necessarily maximizing profits.[4] At CHSL, decisions concerning user fees have reflected all three motivations, and outcomes have indeed given librarians clues for further refinement of the service system. No matter which of several possible economic models might be applied to the question of fees for service, the overall rationale for specific fees has been that the individuals who benefit should pay: the "benefits-received" principle. Focus has been on evolving fair unit fees for transactions in addition to moderate fixed dues for access to the Library's collections. Such "unbundling" of charges has been seen in the new strategy for charging at OCLC, inc., for 1984/85, which now has separate fees for such activities as "display of holdings" and "display of union lists."

ECONOMIES OF SCALE VERSUS CONGESTION: DOCUMENT DELIVERY

Overlap between the personal membership in the Cleveland Medical Library Association and the institutional membership as well as relations with the CWRU university population has caused some complexities and problems, especially as mirrored in the document delivery services. Document delivery has been one of the most conspicuous services rendered at CHSL due to its volume. It has tended to reflect charging policies and system problems in a dramatic way. Institutions with CMLA personal members or CWRU faculty on staff were historically given free services for those patrons, including free loans of materials through a well organized delivery system. Area libraries were encouraged by the economics of the system to send absolutely all requests for such individuals to CHSL, eventually creating a "sorcerer's apprentice" situation of sharply increasing demands for document delivery, particularly by the large teaching hospitals containing many physicians who were also CMLA personal members. Some libraries began the policy of purchasing personal CMLA memberships for physicians on staff in order to achieve a cost reduction. A spiral of increasing use and subsequently decreasing system efficiency burdoned the interlibrary loan system. Users in the Cleveland area asked for more and more items readily available among area hospital libraries. Journal circulation at the Allen Library, a historical benefit of CMLA membership, added to the ponderousness of the system since items became "off the shelf" or "in use" and turn around time for requests slowed. Costs of staffing and for processing requests increased. More and more often the item needed was out of the Library.

Readjustment in the document delivery system became necessary in order to increase efficiency and to assure continued provision of moderately priced, rapid interlibrary loans and photocopies to CMLA personal and institutional members. After some study, library staff decided to implement a policy of charges for personal CMLA members whose requests were handled by the hospitals in which they work, and which institutions benefit directly from their work there. Services to CMLA personal members who dealt directly with CHSL were priced at the same cost, but charged to the personal member. The new charges still contain a $1 price reduction for requests hospitals send to CHSL for CMLA personal members or CWRU faculty, but lessen the imbalance by closing the previous gap and cutting down the incentive to send *ALL* such requests to CHSL. A second necessary move involved ceasing journal circulation at the Allen Library to make the periodical collection available continuously. This also conserved the collection which was sustaining damage from the wear and tear of increasing circulation.

The result of the small adjustments to the cost of photocopies, circulation of journals, and the philosophy of billing resulted in dramatic changes toward network effectiveness and overall system improvement in the Cleveland area. Local health care institutions immediately cooperated to provide free loans and photocopies to each other before utilizing the fee-based services at the Resource Library. Although the larger hospitals found they carried an increased lending workload, they have been able to receive equal benefit by borrowing material from other area libraries. Even the very largest hospital library member has been able to borrow heavily as well as lend due to intense cooperation by the group. All institutions found that the slightly increased cost of photocopies over the previously free loans also paid for a dramatically improved turn around time in filling requests at the Resource Library, and for an additional improvement in fill rate. Less of the collection is out of service in the hands of other users. The readjustment of the document delivery system and the increased cooperation in the Cleveland area have met with great satisfaction among the large proportion of libraries; the smallest libraries which cannot handle the workload are avoided by requesters as a courtesy. All local network libraries have realized a great savings from the cooperative effort, and the remaining quantity of requests provides greater cost recovery for CHSL. The experience with the document delivery system emphasizes the potential complexity of overlapping memberships and the importance of dealing with situations of charging in terms of the larger network implications.

CONCLUSIONS

Using the somewhat complicated fee-for-service system described, the Cleveland Health Sciences Library has defined its "primary" clientele and its role in the local, regional and national library communities. Who is served is identified somewhat uniquely, perhaps, from other libraries due to the historical conditions which have carried into the present. Nevertheless, basic principles of adaptation of services to special needs, use of fixed dues plus unit transaction fees, attention to cost effectiveness of specific services, strategic systems adjustment, and a continuing desire to price services as reasonably as possible allows the Library to generate about 15 percent of its total budget from dues and service fees. For both institutional and personal membership services the Library uses a combination of fixed dues and transaction fees which has helped broaden the base of support. Through marketing of services beyond traditional user populations, CHSL has created a very satisfactory dual membership system in addition to its CWRU user population.

NOTES

1. Fingulin, Jean A. "The Cleveland Medical Library Association." *Bulletin of the Cleveland Medical Library* 22 (October 1976):93–103.

2. Cheshier, Robert G. "Fees for Service in Medical Library Networks." *Bulletin of the Medical Library Association* 60 (April 1972):325–32.

3. Casper, Cheryl A. *Library Pricing Models and Information Requirements: A Case Study.* Ph.D. Cleveland, OH: CWRU, Dept. of Economics, 1975.

4. Casper, Cheryl A. "Estimation of the Demand for Library Services; Draft Final Report, NSF Grant DSI 77-17634. Kent, OH: N.P. 1977, pp. 2–17.

Implementing and Managing
a Fee-Based Information Service
in an Academic Library

John W. Beecher

ABSTRACT. The processes of implementation and management of a fee-based information service in a publicly supported
academic library are examined, based on experiences with fee-
paying clientele anxious for efficient, convenient and flexible
delivery of information. Several ideas for possible future fee-
based services are explored. Attention is focused also on re-
thinking the role of the information professional and the value
of the services and expertise offered information consumers.

In April 1983, the St. Paul Campus Libraries of the University of Minnesota initiated a fee-based information service
called BASIS (Biological and Agricultural Sciences Information Service). The implementation of this service was precipi-
tated by recognized information needs of a secondary, i.e.,
non-University, clientele capable of paying for effective delivery of information available within the Library's agricultural
sciences collections. This article explores some of the basic
concerns associated with establishing and managing a fee-
based information service within the parameters of a publicly
supported academic institution.

THE DECISION TO ESTABLISH A FEE-BASED
INFORMATION SERVICE

Two highly integrated factors must be given prime consideration when initially exploring the possibility of establishing

John W. Beecher is Head of Public Services, St. Paul Campus Libraries, University of Minnesota, and was previously Agricultural Librarian at the University of
Illinois, Urbana-Champaign. He received his M.L.S. from the University of Illinois.

a fee-based information service: what is the scope or range of subject information available for the proposed service to offer clientele, and what is the size and composition of the potential clientele for information within these subject areas?

In the case of the St. Paul Campus Libraries, the nature of the collection circumscribed available services to the subject areas of agriculture and the related biological sciences. BASIS was initially conceived as a means of satisfying the agriculture-related information needs of businesses, industries and governmental agencies in the Minneapolis/St. Paul and surrounding areas. However, it readily became evident there existed a much wider clientele from a much broader geographical area interested in the services proposed. Also, this potential clientele was willing to pay substantial fees for quick, convenient and confidential delivery of information services. Although the fee-based services described here were developed to serve the needs of secondary clientele, it should be noted that the services are available to primary clientele wishing to make use of them.

During initial planning, there existed considerable concern among the Library's staff regarding the ability of an academic library to compete successfully with information brokers from the private sector. However, it must be realized that many indirect costs—such as rents, utilities, capital investments in major equipment—are provided by the parent institution. Access to the collections, photocopy equipment and delivery services is generally immediate, adding to the potential for quick and efficient services. Also, the academic library probably has a diversified professional and support staff on board, familiar with the idiosyncrasies of the collection and the library itself, adding to the potential for effective services. Based on these factors, most academic libraries can probably provide efficient delivery of fee-based services at cheaper rates than most private enterprises could afford to offer. The potential undoubtedly exists in most academic libraries to provide a wide array of fee-based services, perhaps more services than the majority of information brokers from the private sector could consider offering.

Once the two primary and interdependent factors—available subject areas and potential clientele—are explored and determined favorable for establishing a fee-based information service, attention shifts to examining more variable factors such as: possible services to be offered; potential impacts on current operations, policies, and staffing patterns; and projected funding needs and competitive fee structures.

CONCEPTUALIZING SERVICES AND ESTABLISHING POLICIES

The immediate situation faced in St. Paul was that the ever-increasing demands for library services by the secondary users were seriously hampering the staff's ability to meet the needs of the primary clientele (faculty, students and staff of the University). Decreasing real dollars budgeted to publicly supported libraries effectively results in decreasing quality and quantity of services available to all users—primary or secondary. Serving the needs of the secondary clientele was generating a certain amount of good will, but no income that could be used directly to support or expand current services for either primary or secondary users. Limits had to be established regarding services to the secondary clientele or such services had to be supported by direct charges. Of these alternatives, the latter seemed the more constructive. Through a synergistic relationship, a fee-based information service offers alternative means of generating revenues to contribute positively to the continued development and vitality of a major research library.

Understanding that it is important to maintain good community relations, but that it is also important to use discretion in dispensing a major resource—the Library staff's time and expertise—policies regarding the extent of free services to be offered secondary clientele had to be established. The Library staff continues to provide the following services gratis to secondary clientele: searching in two appropriate major indexing services (including those online); and/or searching relevant journals or other resources with a limit of no more than ten minutes of staff time per request. If satisfactory service can be provided using any one or a combination of the above guidelines, staff assistance is provided to all users. The reference interview usually tends to identify the user's affiliation. The source of a telephone inquiry is usually even more easily identified; almost all requests require a return call—and the name or telephone number generally indicates the affiliation of the caller. If the request cannot be answered satisfactorily using the established guidelines, secondary clientele are told (1) they may continue to use the resources themselves, or (2) continued assistance is available for a fee, i.e., BASIS.

Establishing a fee-based information service during times of major institutional retrenchments meant significant funds were not readily forthcoming to hire additional clerical or professional staff—especially given the possibility that sufficient demand to support a fee-for-service operation may not have existed. Therefore, the aid and support of the current staff was enlisted.

Personnel familiar with the Library's collections and other resources were identified to provide services for various aspects of the proposed fee-based service. The interlibrary loan department was made the home of BASIS, and the head of interlibrary loan was designated coordinator of all document delivery services: interlibrary loan, a USDA document delivery service for which the Library has a regional-center contract, a paging and photocopy service for University personnel, and the new fee-based information service for secondary clientele. A minimal amount of student wage funds were allocated to this expanded operation for paging and photocopying. Professional librarians were encouraged to provide reference services for the new venture since the BASIS staff would be responsible for most verification and paging operations throughout the St. Paul Campus Libraries—thereby freeing departmental support staffs for other operations within their respective units.

Throughout planning to meet the service demands of a fee-paying but secondary clientele, considerable attention had to be devoted to maintaining or improving the current level of services to the Library's primary clientele. These concerns focus attention on management's responsibility to review, update, and establish necessary procedural and policy statements. Written policies and the parameters of services to be offered have to be provided, plus rationale and consistent policies regarding available services. It is very important to establish—in writing—that the fee-based services are offered with no guarantee of results. Although offering the Library staff's time and expertise to retrieve information relevant to a client's inquiry, the services of BASIS do not include actual interpretations, or written analysis or opinions of the supplied information or materials. A written statement was drafted that BASIS is not liable for accuracy or thoroughness of the information and materials provided. Also, University counsel was consulted regarding "fair use" and the need for a copyright disclaimer statement.

Establishing BASIS also resulted in updating circulation, recall and fine policies, reviewing record keeping procedures for copyright purposes, and reaffirming established collection development statements. There was considerable concern expressed by bibliographers that acquisitions funds would be used for collecting in areas outside the scope of our primary-user demands; in short, there was an assumption that a fee-based service implies collection development obligations. Policy statements had to be developed to insure that collection development policies, already in effect for all major subject areas of the St. Paul Campus Libraries, would not be altered to satisfy the needs of the secondary clientele. Also, although BASIS is designed primarily to provide access to the Library's collections, it was determined that interlibrary loan services would be used for items not available on campus but deemed within the scope of current subject coverage.

The concept of fee-based information has a history of creating controversy within the library profession.[1,2] There still exists a sense among some librarians that a tax-supported institution should offer all library services "free." However, many of today's users already expect to pay for certain services. One example is photocopy—often a self-service operation and certainly a service that requires no use of the professional skills available within a library. The same is true of various coin-operated services, such as typewriters and calculators. Can coin-operated microcomputers be far away? Database searching services, requiring certain professional skills, are generally offered on a fee-for-service basis, even when subsidized with library funds. All of this supports the idea that many library users recognize the need for direct charges to maintain, expand and render special library services, especially if these services include the use of some level of staff expertise. Charges for specialized services effectively and efficiently developed to deliver information to meet a client's particular needs is recognized as a reasonable proposition by almost all users.

ESTABLISHING A "VALUE" FOR A FEE-BASED INFORMATION SERVICE

John Naisbitt in *Megatrends*[3] states that, "Information is an economic entity that people are willing to pay for; the value is determined by what people are asked—and willing—to pay." This underscores an important principle for the manager of an information service—the librarian or information professional possesses an extremely marketable skill. James B. Dodd,[4] in a paper presented at the 1982 Conference on Fee Based Research in College and University Libraries, states: "We do the profession a disserve when we don't charge for certain services. We do an even greater disserve when we charge a token fee which seems to indicate that the services are worth something but not a whole lot."

BASIS is an information service founded on a two-fold fee-based approach; it sells a service—expertise in accessing (but not interpreting) relevant information, rendered by the professional staff and charged on a per-hour basis; and it sells a product—document delivery, handled by the support staff and charged on a per-item basis. Document delivery services currently available for a per-item fee include photocopies or loans of materials from the collections or obtained through interlibrary loan, as well as verification of incomplete or elusive citations. Rush service is also available at a premium fee per item. Professional services available for a per-hour fee (plus direct costs) include reference services relative to the subject areas of the collections, plus online as well as manual bibliographic searching. Current awareness services are also available for an annual fee plus direct costs.

FEE-BASED SERVICES IN AN AGE OF ELECTRONICS

The future of a fee-based information service such as BASIS—approximately 92 percent of income during the first fiscal year was generated by the hard-copy document delivery service—may be severely limited by the continuing development of affordable electronic communications systems. However, such communications developments also will lead to growing demands for access to information in appropriate formats delivered within cost-effective time frames. And there will exist—perhaps more so tomorrow than today—a need for information professionals to service such demands.

Meanwhile, libraries continue their role as one of the places people depend on for access to information. In addition to the printed resources, libraries currently provide terminals needed to access an ever-growing number of electronic resources; and, more importantly, librarians provide the expertise needed to exploit these resources most effectively. However, as electronic resources continue to gain importance and hard copy resources diminish, as terminals become more commonplace in offices and homes, and as individual researchers become more familiar and comfortable with the use of these online resources, the need to visit libraries will rapidly diminish.[5] A fee-based service provides a vehicle for expanding information services to a growing but less library-oriented clientele, thereby offering a means for information professionals to establish their worth (or value) to seekers of information.

Obviously, information professionals can—today as well as tomorrow—offer training seminars, institutes and workshops to keep clients up to date regarding new sources of information. Another fee-based role for information professionals is that of consultant, ranging from such basic services as pointing users in the direction of resources most appropriate for solving their particular information needs, to training clients in accessing electronic resources or actually searching sources (manual or online) that are unfamiliar to the user. The repackaging of information also offers opportunities for information professionals to demonstrate their expertise, for example, assisting researchers in the organization of personal electronic files or the construction of user-interest profiles for use with online SDI services. Subject specialists have the opportunity to function as experts providing "information analysis," such as synthesizing the results of searches in several sources and presenting evaluated and selective results to the client. Information professionals, especially subject specialists, have opportunities to become entrepreneurs, perhaps building databases or creating public information files for use on cable TV. All of these services, and undoubtedly many others, are quite feasible and encouraged within the environment of a fee-based information service. The potentials are almost limitless—and largely unexplored.

Richard DeGennaro[6] recently stated that fee-based information services "pose no threat to libraries. . . , they supplement them by filling needs and demands that publicly supported libraries cannot and should not try to meet—providing special and expensive services to business, professional, and other users who can afford them." Moreover, as part of the process described here, professional librarians as a group are changing their attitudes about themselves, the profession of librarianship, and their perceptions of the clientele served.[7] Also, and perhaps most importantly, fee-based information services play a significant role in helping librarians rethink their relationship with clientele and reconsider the value (or value-added) of their work and the services provided.

REFERENCES

1. "Moon Selects Target: U.S. Information Policy," *American Libraries* 8 (July/August 1977):381.

2. "The Prostitution of Information Fees for Service," *American Libraries* 8 (March 1977):139.

3. Naisbitt, John. *Megatrends: Ten New Directions Transforming Our Lives.* New York: Warner Books, Inc., 1982.

4. Dodd, James Beaupre. "In's and Out's of Charging for Research Services." In: *Conference on Fee Based Research in College and University Libraries.* Greenvale, N.Y.: Center for Business Research, C.W. Post Center, Long Island University, 1983, pp. 20–34.

5. Lancaster, F.W., and Beecher, John W. "Agricultural Librarianship and Documentation as a Profession." In: *Agricultural Information to Hasten Development: Proceedings of the Sixth World Congress of Agricultural Librarians and Documentalists held at the Philippine International Convention Center, Manila, Philippines, 3–7 March 1980.* (1981):197–210.

6. DeGennaro, Richard. "Libraries, Technology, and the Information Marketplace." *Library Journal* 107 (1 June 1982):1045–1054.

7. Smith, Eldred R. "Fees for Service: Rationale and Management Decisions." Paper presented at the *Twentieth Century Agricultural Science Symposium, National Agricultural Library, October 22, 1982.* Unpublished proceedings.

SELECTED BIBLIOGRAPHY

Evans, G. Edward. *Management Techniques for Librarians.* 2nd edition. New York, N.Y.: Academic Press, 1983.

Lancaster, F.W. *Libraries and Librarians in an Age of Electronics.* Arlington, VA: Information Resources Press, 1982.

Martell, Charles R., Jr. *The Client-Centered Academic Library; An Organizational Model.* Westport, CT: Greenwood Press, 1983.

Reid, Richard C. "Fee-Based Services and Collection Development in an Academic Library." *Drexel Library Quarterly* 19 (Fall 1983):54–67.

Ungarelli, Donald, and Grant, Mary McNierney. "A Fee-Based Model: Administrative Considerations in an Academic Library." *Drexel Library Quarterly* 19 (Fall 1983):4–12.

Information Brokering M & S Style

Michal A. Stefanacci
Michele I. Martin

ABSTRACT. The typical services provided by information brokers and their role within the information framework are discussed. A case history of a moderately successful information brokerage business, Martin & Stefanacci Associates, is provided.

INTRODUCTION

Much has been written about fee-based information services, and information brokers in particular, since the genre first surfaced in the mid-1970s. The growth of these services is due to a large extent to the following factors:[1]

1. The ever increasing size and complexity of the information industry itself.
2. Decreasing costs of online searching and the increasing use of publicly available databases by a greater number of searchers, professional and amateur alike.
3. Cutbacks in public sector spending.
4. Increased awareness by companies and other organizations of the value of information.
5. Growing support for small business.

The success of these private ventures is significantly related to what Maxine Davis delineates as the characteristics necessary for freelancing.[2] Among the required attributes she includes: an understanding of the power of information; the ability to interpret accurately the actual needs of the client; adapt-ability

---

Michal A. Stefanacci is an Information Consultant, 2766 Stevens Summit, Columbia, PA 17512. She received her M.S.L.S. from Drexel University. Michele I. Martin is Research Director, The Information Link, 1636 Sunset Avenue, Lancaster, PA 17601. She received her M.S.L.S. from Villanova University.

to constantly changing situations; the ability to interpret, synthesize, and repackage information; skill in communicating and working with non-library-oriented individuals; business expertise and administrative ability; ability to empathize with the client; and finally, the ability to work independently.

In the following article, the services and role of information brokers in general will be defined. Additionally, a case history of a moderately successful information brokerage business, Martin and Stefanacci Associates, will be presented.

INFORMATION BROKERS DEFINED

Patricia Schick has described the information broker as an unknown type of service—one which "defies a 30 second promo or a snappy jingle."[3] Essentially, and simply, the information broker fills the gap between the information provider and the information user. The information broker utilizes his research skills and expertise in knowing the fastest and most efficient retrieval channels to supply relevant information, on demand, rapidly and cost effectively.

Most information brokerage services started as one or two-person businesses, some on a part-time basis while the owners held other full-time jobs. Many were started by corporate librarians, who saw a need for individualized research. To no one's great surprise the largest concentration of information brokers is in New York and California. The major metropolitan areas of Colorado, New Jersey, Massachusetts, Maryland, Illinois, Pennsylvania, Virginia, and Washington, D.C. also are areas of heavy brokering activity.[1] For every large, well-established information-on-demand organization in the United States, there are at least ten other small one or two-person operations.[4]

The major problems faced by the smaller brokerages are: the need to educate, and cost of educating, the market; and the need to establish pricing structures for services and products which will be profitable and competitive. To be successful, brokerage firm owners must exhibit business sense combined with careful control of cash flow and overheads. Excellent contacts within as well as outside the information industry and the development of at least one unique service or product (at least in the immediate geographic area) are important factors. Finally, the ability to talk as an equal with senior managers and executives is essential.[1]

Typical Services

The major service of the information broker is to provide information on request. Clients usually come from business, industry, government, and the social services. Less often a request may come from the academic environment, such as a student researching a term paper or a college or university faculty member.

Being able to provide specialized information quickly via computer databases is probably the biggest selling point for the information broker. In fact, online searching appears to be the catalyst for the number of information brokerages currently in operation.[1] The growth of available databases is no less than phenomenal. In 1976 there were a total of 486 databases; by 1980 that number had grown to 1400, and latest data indicate there are as many as 2014 databases now online.[5,6] In addition to retrospective literature searching, most brokers also provide current awareness services custom-tailored to the needs of their clients.

Document delivery is another service of major importance. Some brokerage firms, like Information-on-Demand, specialize in document delivery. Document retrieval is generally not limited to the results of an online or manual information search. Most firms will retrieve any document requested by the client.

Other services offered may vary from broker to broker, but in general include:[7]

—Indexing
—Thesaurus development
—Directory compilation
—Library organization
—Abstracting
—Conducting training sessions
—Translating
—Cataloging and classification of library collections
—Analysis, interpretation or presentation of reports and studies custom-tailored to clients' needs

Typical Structure

The typical structure of an information brokerage firm is the same as in any other business, based on the pyramid format. However, it adds to its resources by employing an interconnecting network of databases, marketing and advertising experts, librarians, and consultants.

Since very few information brokerages are large operations, most rely heavily on part-time staff. Many, regardless of size, have a network of "stringers" or "field investigators" who locate and retrieve documents in libraries and information centers around the world. A computer programmer might be retained to help write the software for an in-house indexing system. Marketing, advertising, and public relations specialists are often utilized on a retainer basis to enhance the overall business capability. Consultants, who may be other free-lance librarians or brokers, are used on a part-time basis as needed. For instance, a client needs information relating to a lawsuit concerning a defect in medical equipment. A consultant might be contacted for research in any one of these fields: medicine, law, technical or patent data.

Role Within the Total Information Service Framework

A surprising number of libraries and other organizations that already have access to information technology make use of private information-on-demand services.[8] There are a number of reasons for this. In many cases deteriorating budgets and personnel cuts have resulted in the curtailment of needed or expected services. Oftentimes, employment of an outside source can reinstate a service at a fraction of the cost. In addition, the increase in the volume of information materials available to and desired by patrons, and the advent of new technology into information transfer processes have overloaded an already reduced staff. A temporary work overload or a one-time request for information outside the scope of in-house specialization can be circumvented by using the services of an information broker.

Two other factors significantly influence the use, by libraries, of professional services from private organizations. First, many libraries have begun to recognize that frequently used services and products should be handled in-house. On the other hand, infrequently used ones can be provided most efficiently and cost effectively by outside organizations or by sharing resources.[9] Secondly, information managers in traditional settings do not generally have the time to provide in-depth reference help, even to their primary clients.[3] The information broker, particularly the smaller one, is geared to act as a "personal research assistant" and can devote the time and energy necessary to complete a comprehensive or lengthy project.

Confidentiality, especially in industry and the legal profession, is often a prime factor in employing an outside force. By working through an intermediary, the requester of the information remains anonymous and the integrity of current cases or future projects or ventures is maintained. The fast turn-around time promoted by private information-on-demand services in also of significant importance to a number of clients, both institutional and individual. Additionally, small companies or other organizations often need "one-time" service for organizing files or collections, indexing or abstracting, bibliographic research for special projects, compilation of directories, or general consulting.[9]

Individuals are increasingly utilizing the services of brokers, once the mental block against fee-based services is overcome and the realization dawns that personal and thorough service is rendered. Time and geographic constraints also lead more individuals to the information broker's door, even in the midst of the "computer on everyone's desk" phenomenon that is sweeping the nation. As higher management continues to recognize that information is a valuable, tangible resource, and encourages staff to make more effective use of that information, the role of the broker in filling the gap between services available and user needs will continue to expand.

Dennis Lewis[6] predicted in 1980 that the information broker would come of age between 1980 and 1995, and that information brokering would develop into a highly profitable sphere of commercial activity. His foresight already has been proven by the success of so many private services. Mr. Lewis also contended that such growth will probably abate as the compatibility of systems renders the entire universe of organized knowledge available to the less sophisticated searcher. Only time will tell if this hypothesis, too, proves to be correct.

MARTIN & STEFANACCI ASSOCIATES

Background

Martin & Stefanacci Associates was started, like most other information brokerages, by two experienced, special librarians who saw a need to provide an information service to business, industry, and professionals. A lack of experience in owning a business necessitated initial research of small businesses in general, including attendance at Small Business Administration workshops with the intention of expanding business knowledge and exploring possible options. Based on previous work experience in a corporate setting or academic environment, our point of view had to be adjusted to a more personal perspective.

At the same time, a second research and planning stage evolved, with the objective of gathering information to help answer the following questions. First, what was the best structure for the business? Should it be operated as a partnership and was it necessary to incorporate, or should one person own the business and the other be an employee? Next, what types of services could be offered, what information sources were available to the business, and how should the services be priced? The local market had to be identified along with the marketing strategy. Also, immediate equipment needs had to be determined; and last, but certainly not least, the financial resources available to the business had to be assessed. Most decisions regarding these questions were made after a careful study of similar services, and after determining the availability and accessibility of information sources.

After evaluating the public and private financial assistance available at that time, the decision was made to finance the business ourselves. By pooling the resources of the owners, the business could remain solvent for at least one year. Initially, the largest expense was equipment. A used Texas Instrument Silent 700 printer terminal (TI 745 portable) and two telephones were purchased. The second largest expense was the design of the business logo and the printing of stationery, envelopes, and business cards. Less costly was the purchase of user manuals and database thesauri. Office expenses and overhead were kept to a minimum by working from the homes of the owners.

A simple partnership was formed. Martin & Stefanacci Associates (M&S) became official in September 1980 when a business partnership was filed with the IRS.

To begin, services provided by M&S were limited to literature searching (not necessarily online), document delivery, and current awareness. DIALOG was the primary online information source, and the resources of several large, academic libraries, medical libraries, and a number of special libraries in the local area provided the primary access for document delivery.

Since there were no other information brokers in the immediate geographic area, the partnership's services were priced so as to be comparable to other small information brokers, but less than large firms which were potentially providing services to organizations in the same geographic area. A decision was made to contact medium to large industry; professional individuals, such as attorneys, doctors, dentists, and consultants; marketing and advertising agencies; libraries; and organizations. The partnership's primary market was the five-county area surrounding Lancaster, Pennsylvania. Direct mail was selected as the method for initial contact with possible clients and a letter was created describing the services offered by M&S. After the initial contact, follow-up was made with a phone call. Mailing lists were developed from directories that were readily available. Over time, it has been found that those directories which supply a contact name or list of officer names and/or names of those in management positions are, by far, the best to use. Possibly the hardest part of any selling job is finding the right person to talk to in a company or business.

At the outset a lack of organization and structure proved to be a major problem. Initially, since this was a partnership, everything was done together. Quickly, the potential of dividing the work load became apparent. There were certain tasks which one partner enjoyed more than the other or was simply better at than the other. These tasks were divided as evenly as possible so that one partner was able to work most of the time at a job regardless of whether the time suited the other partner. Outside consultants or other librarians were seldom used to provide any of the actual services, although sometimes contacts in the field were very helpful in suggesting possible sources of information.

Services

Martin & Stefanacci Associates, like the majority of information brokers, currently offers a wide range of services, from bibliographic research to general consulting. Each request for information is treated as comprehensively as possible. Of course, all information sources are fully documented. During the past three years the partnership has expanded its online resources to include the databases offered through Infoline, BRS, Dow Jones, and Vu/Text in addition to DIALOG.

By virtue of repetition more than anything else, M&S has developed expertise in a few key areas. The Research and Development (R&D) departments of several companies in the food industry frequently request technological information from M&S to support current projects. By working closely with the individuals involved in the actual research, it is possible to gain a clear understanding of the information needed and the form that the information should take. For example, a search of the patent literature may be necessary to identify patents for a certain piece of industrial equipment, or patents held by a particular company.

Advertising agencies and marketing consultants ask for background technological and marketing information—sort of a first step in developing a new account. An overview of the results of previously conducted studies allows the agency or consultant to plan its/his own strategy without duplicating work already done.

Some of the partnership's heaviest users are lawyers engaged in personal injury litigation. Their need for medical and technical information, supported by full-text documents, is astronomical. Local medical libraries offer limited fee-based search services to outside patrons, usually consisting of a

MEDLINE search and/or document delivery. Lawyers know this and have relied for years on what help the local medical librarian could provide. However, with the number of online databases available growing daily and the subsequent exponential increase in the number of references cited and requested, the medical librarian is lucky to keep ahead of in-house information needs, let alone those of "outsiders." Many of M&S's clients in the legal profession have been direct referrals from medical librarians who cannot devote the time necessary to gather all the information requested.

A significant number of "expert witness" searches are requested by clients. These are not searches for expert witnesses, but rather searches for biographical information about or references to literature published by individuals identified by counsel to testify as "experts" in a given court case. Many of the medical information requests which are received by M&S require extensive manual as well as online research. Long-distance telephone calls, perusal of medical supply catalogs, verification of names and addresses, and document delivery are typical of the comprehensive service provided by Martin & Stefanacci Associates. M&S, because of its specialized services, is able to give more individualized attention to this type of request.

Several clients have requested help in designing space for an in-house library. Library procedures manuals have recently become a forte of the business. Instrumental in locating qualified information professionals for newly created library positions has been a network of professional colleagues.

The current awareness services provided by M&S vary in frequency, content and format, depending upon the nature of the information and the requirements of the user. At least one client receives weekly updates on specified topics and in a custom tailored format via an electronic mail system.

One of the newest services offered by M&S is the development of a core package. An analysis of requests led to the realization that similar information was frequently being provided to different clients. The topic might change, but the type of data needed followed a pattern. Therefore, a package was designed which included a set of reliable sources to be searched for each request. The client knows beforehand exactly what information is potentially available and the sources from which it is generated.

Pricing

The matter of pricing is of crucial importance in any business, for if the pricing strategy is not viable, the business will fail.[10] Many pricing models are currently employed by information brokers and no dominant method prevails. Among the more commonly employed forms are: invoice upon completion, deposit accounts, and retainer or subscription fees. Martin & Stefanacci Associates uses a combination of invoice and retainer/subscription fee. Most accounts are invoiced upon completion of each project. A retainer fee of 25 percent of the total estimated cost is generally required for long-term research or consulting projects, with additional remuneration designated for each stage of completion. Current awareness services are provided on a subscription basis.

An emphasis on competent personal service at reasonable cost has been and continues to be the key to success for M&S. People like to know the people with whom they are dealing and we do become each client's "personal assistant."

Marketing

Much depends upon the skill with which information services are marketed.[10] Personal contact, direct mail, referrals from colleagues or satisfied customers, and advertisements placed in telephone directories, business periodicals and through public relations channels are the most widely used techniques. To whom these services are marketed is also of paramount importance, and the identification of this market is a continual and constantly changing process. The importance of this process to the success of the business cannot be overemphasized.

Several marketing techniques have proven effective for M&S. Direct referral from current clients or professional colleagues is by far the most effective. Personal contact, either through "cold calls" or semi-formal discussions at business or professional gatherings generates a large percentage of client interest and subsequent contracts. The partners spend considerable time and energy being visible.

A direct mail campaign is an effective way to contact a large target audience quickly. A simple brochure, clearly and cleverly designed to promote the broker's services, is essential. A "personal" cover letter and other inserts, such as a reply card, also are beneficial. Unless a broker has a large marketing staff (most don't), a follow-up call to each direct mail recipient is impossible. The trick is to segment the mailing list into major areas and identify a few prime possibilities from each segment. A call is then placed to each of these candidates in order to discuss services in further detail. Marketing is more often than not an exercise in educating the potential client. Meeting this challenge successfully involves hard work and patience.

DEVELOPMENTAL CHANGES WITHIN MARTIN & STEFANACCI ASSOCIATES

Areas of Responsibility

As noted earlier in discussing the beginning of Martin & Stefanacci Associates, rather than work together on everything, tasks were divided so that each partner could work separately. As the business progressed the division of tasks was refined to the division of actual areas of responsibility. One partner became totally responsible for the marketing function and current awareness updates. The other took over the research function, which included most literature searching, and all document delivery. Each, of course, provides backup for the other when necessary and a helping hand when needed.

An important area of responsibility, and one which involves both partners, is keeping current professionally. This is no easy task especially in the areas of online databases, computers, and the electronic offices of today. Reading, seminars, conferences, and workshops are all work-related activities which do not show tangible dollar results but are very necessary to the business.

The Changing Scene

Technological advances in information storage, retrieval and transfer have definitely modified our methods of providing information during the past three years. Electronic mail has transformed document delivery for the business. Most references can now be verified and requested online, thus expediting the delivery of full-text articles to the client. The ability to combine the storage and editing capabilities of the personal computer with electronic mail has made it possible to reformat and enhance information and then send it directly to a client. With the growing number of full-text databases and the ever increasing size of all databases, the ability to download information for later editing also has proven valuable.

At the other end of the spectrum of changes, a growing concern over ethics in information brokering has forced all brokers to take a hard look at the methods used to gather information and at the basic question of who actually owns the information obtained. M&S, like most brokers, considers that information already in the public domain belongs to everyone and that service, not information, is being sold. It does seem to be a difficult concept for some to grasp.

FUTURE DIRECTIONS AND PLANNING

As in all businesses, goals must be set. Future plans for Martin & Stefanacci Associates include: expansion of the geographical area served; development of subject-specific and/or market-specific services; distribution of a regular newsletter to current and potential clients; and an increase in the number of online databases offered. Keeping abreast of and utilizing new technology of potential benefit to Martin & Stefanacci and our clients continues to be a major goal.

REFERENCES

1. White, Martin S. *Information Brokering Services in U.S.A.: Report of a Study Trip, April/May 1979.* London: NPM Information Services Ltd., 1981.
2. "Information Brokers: Who, What, Why, How." *Bulletin of the American Society for Information Science* 2 (February 1976):11–20.
3. Schick, Patricia. "The Information Company." In: *Proceedings of the Fifth Canadian Conference on Information Science, Ottawa, May 15–18, 1977.* Ottawa: Canadian Association for Information Science, 1977, pp. 201–6.
4. Bellomy, F. "The Information Brokerage Scene in America." In: *Proceedings of the 1st International Online Information Meeting, London, December 13–15, 1977.* New York: Learned Information, 1977, pp. 215–23.

5. *Directory of Online Databases, 1984 Supplement.* Santa Monica, Ca.: Cuadra Associates, Inc., 1984.

6. Lewis, Dennis A. "Today's Challenge—Tomorrow's Choice: Change or Be Changed or the Doomsday Scenario Mk2." *Journal of Information Science* 2 (September 1980):59–74.

7. Ferguson, Patricia. "Chronicles of an Information Company." *Online Review* 1 (March 1977):39–42.

8. Schick, Renee, and Levy, Alix C. "On-Demand Information Services." In: Simora, Filornena, ed. *Bowker Annual of Library & Book Trade Information.* New York: R.R. Bowker Co., 1980, pp. 66–9.

9. Creager, William A., and King, Donald W. "Professional Services Provided to Libraries and Information Centers by Private Sector Organizations." In: O'Hare, Joanne, ed., *Bowker Annual of Library & Book Trade Information.* New York: R.R. Bowker Co., 1983, pp. 48–55.

10. Archer, Mary Ann E. "The 'Make or Buy' Decision: Five Main Points to Consider." *Online* 2 (July 1978):24–5.

ADDITIONAL REFERENCES

Clayton, Audrey, and Nisenoff, N. "Changes in Information Delivery Systems Over the Next Two Decades." In: *Proceedings of the 1st International Online Meeting, London, December 13–15, 1977.* New York: Learned Information, 1977, pp. 17–25.

Kostrewski, B.J., and Oppenheim, Charles. "Ethics in Information Science." *Journal of Information Science* 1 (January 1980):277–83.

Stefanacci, Michal A., and Martin, Michele I. "Getting a Handle on Information Retrieval." In: Pennsylvania Manufacturing Confectioners' Association. *Proceedings of the Thirty-seventh Annual Production Conference, April 26–28, 1983.* Drexel Hill, Pa.: 1983, pp. 74–5.

Warnken, Kelly. *The Information Brokers: How to Start and Operate Your Own Fee-Based Service.* New York: R.R. Bowker Co., 1981.

V. ANNOTATED BIBLIOGRAPHY

Cost Accounting, Marketing, and Fee-Based Services: An Annotated Bibliography

M. Sandra Wood

This bibliography is intended to bring together key literature related to cost analysis, cost recovery and marketing library reference and fee-based information services. Although the emphasis of this supplement is on health sciences libraries, it is necessary to draw on the literature about all types of libraries and from business sources to achieve an overall picture. The literature published for public, special, and academic libraries is interrelated. For example, the fee-versus-free issue, which has special implications for public libraries, is relevant to the overall perspective of costs and fee structures in special or academic libraries. Library marketing literature, in particular, draws heavily from the business literature; especially relevant is marketing in non-profit organizations and marketing of services.

Entries for this bibliography have been selected from *Library Literature* and *Business Periodicals Index,* and from a variety of bibliographies found in books and journal articles; all of the items have been examined by the author. The majority of entries were published from 1975 to September 1984; several items from 1970 to 1974 were selected for inclusion based either on their relevance to health sciences libraries or

M. Sandra Wood is Head, Reference, The George T. Harrell Library, The Milton S. Hershey Medical Center, The Pennsylvania State University, Hershey, PA 17033. She received an M.L.S. from Indiana University and an M.L.S. from the University of Maryland

on their general applicability (e.g., a review article). The bibliography places an emphasis on online searching because it is one service which, from the beginning, has been at the heart of the fee-for-service issue. While it was not possible to be complete, it is hoped that a majority of the most relevant literature is included. In particular, materials from the business literature are highly selective; for example, the literature on marketing of nonprofit organizations and services is extensive, and only highly selected items are included here. Additionally, only a sampling of literature on information brokers is included because of their relationship to fee-based services in libraries; the primary focus, however, is on business aspects of reference information services in libraries.

Certain items were specifically excluded from this bibliography either due to lack of availability or to the brevity of the item—for example, letters to the editor and meeting proceedings. Further information can be found in proceedings such as the National Online meetings and *ASLIB Proceedings*. In the case of the free-versus-fee issue, which has been extensively debated in journals such as *Library Journal*, representative editorials have been included.

The bibliography is divided into six areas: general sources, which includes both overviews and items which cover more than one subject area; cost analysis; cost recovery; marketing; fee-based services; and information brokers. Entries within each subject area are then listed alphabetically by author. Annotations for each entry provide a synopsis of the article or book.

GENERAL SOURCES

Atherton, Pauline, and Christian, Roger W. *Librarians and Online Services.* White Plains, N.Y.: Knowledge Industry Publications, Inc., 1977.

Atherton and Christian describe basic considerations necessary for establishing and managing online search services. Chapters include "Financial Considerations" and "Marketing and Promotion."

Braunstein, Yale M. "Costs and Benefits of Library Information: The User Point of View." *Library Trends* 28 (Summer 1979):79–87.

Information has value in itself, but the medium for obtaining information also has value. Similarly, the costs of using a library can be borne not only by the library itself, but by the user (private costs). Pricing has a variety of implications for both the library and the user as far as a cost/benefit relationship. This is part of a thematic issue on "The Economics of Academic Libraries."

Cheshier, Robert G. "Providing Library Services in a Time of Fiscal Crisis: Alternatives." *Bulletin of the Medical Library Association* 65 (October 1977): 419–24.

Fee-for-service (primarily document delivery) is one alternative mentioned by Cheshier in attempting to match costs to services.

De Gennaro, Richard. "Libraries, Technology, and the Information Marketplace." *Library Journal* 107 (June 1, 1982): 1045–54.

De Gennaro states that "libraries are alive and well and adapting to a changing world." In a general discussion about information and the library's role within the new technology, the author warns about believing all predictions about the future, discusses the "paperless society" and Giuliano's manifesto, and discusses interlibrary loan and online services as provided by libraries versus information brokers or other fee services. Libraries will continue to be a vital link between commercial vendors and the users of information.

Fenichel, Carol H., and Hogan, Thomas H. *Online Searching: A Primer*. Marlton, N.J.: Learned Information, Inc., 1981.

Intended as a basic introduction to online searching, this text covers everything from databases and vendors through management of online search services. Of particular interest is the chapter on "Costs and Charging Policies" (pp. 77–83), which gives an overview of the financial considerations in online searching.

Hitchingham, Eileen E. "MEDLINE Use in a University Without a School of Medicine." *Special Libraries* 67 (April 1976):188–94.

This study of MEDLINE use, designed to evaluate search characteristics and user satisfaction, includes unit cost data. Searches were provided free of charge for the study. Both faculty and students "indicated willingness to pay for future searches," with acceptable fees ranging from $2.50 to $50.

Hoover, Ryan E. "Computer Aided Reference Services in the Academic Library; Experiences in Organizing and Operating an Online Reference Service." *Online* 3 (October 1979):28–41.

The organization and operation of Computer-Aided Reference Services at the University of Utah Libraries is described. Hoover presents ten essential aspects to consider in organizing a formal online search unit, including marketing and promotion, and pricing and budgeting.

Hoover, Ryan E., ed. *The Library and Information Manager's Guide to Online Services.* White Plains, N.Y.: Knowledge Industry Publications, Inc., 1980.

Information needed for establishing and maintaining an online search service is presented. Information on vendor costs, contracts and billing is included in the chapter by Alice H. Bahr, "Producers and Vendors of Bibliographic Online Services," pp. 65–96, while Donald T. Hawkins includes a discussion of costing out and charging for online searches in his chapter, "Management of an Online Information Retrieval Service," pp. 97–125. In another chapter by Bahr, "Promotion of Online Services," pp. 161–79, online searching is treated as a special service; promotional tactics include brochures, fliers, press releases, demonstrations, and free searches.

Kibirige, Harry M. *The Information Dilemma; A Critical Analysis of Information Pricing and the Fees Controversy.* Westport, Connecticut: Greenwood Press, 1983. (New Directions in Librarianship, Number 4).

An overview of information technology and the information industry/services of the 1980s is provided. Chapters include "The Information Industry and Market in the United States"; "User Access to Information" (includes the fees controversy); "Pricing Information Services and Products" (includes price theory and cost concepts); and "Information Marketing Research."

Knapp, Sara D., and Schmidt, C. James. "Budgeting to Provide Computer-Based Reference Services: A Case Study." *Journal of Academic Librarianship* 5 (March 1979):9–13.
The imposition of fees to cover the costs of offline printing at SUNY/Albany is discussed, along with the rationale for making the decision. The provision of online searching from 1972 to 1977 as a totally free service is summarized. Estimated direct expenses to be absorbed by the institution for online searching for 1977–78 were $15,600.

Kobelski, Pamela, and Trumbore, Jean. "Student Use of Online Bibliographic Services." *Journal of Academic Librarianship* 4 (March 1978):14–8.
The Morris Library at the University of Delaware received a grant to promote the use of online search services by students. The grant paid half the total charges, while the student paid the other half. The study includes analysis by subsidized and non-subsidized searches for such data as type of user, average search time, and cost to the user; a total cost distribution of searches for subsidized versus non-subsidized searches; user satisfaction, as related to cost of the search and number of citations generated; and frequency of databases searched. Promotional techniques and costing information are discussed.

Lewis, Davis W. "Bringing the Market to Libraries." *Journal of Academic Librarianship* 10 (May 1984):73–6.
A market system based on user subsidies is proposed as a means of making both users and librarians aware of the costs involved in providing services. "Libdollars" would be issued by the library; patrons could use this artifically created money to select and use certain services up to a prespecified quota. The author also addresses performance criteria, incentive systems and internal information systems. This is an excellent article to introduce librarians to the need to be aware of the costs involved in providing services and the need to adopt a market system.

Wax, David M. *A Handbook for the Introduction of On-Line Bibliographic Search Services into Academic Libraries*. Washington, D.C.: Association of Research Libraries, 1976. (Office of University Library Management Studies Occasional Papers. Number Four).

Libraries initiating (and reevaluating) online search services can use this publication as a guide. Included are areas such as staffing, organization, and training. The chapter on user education includes brief information on promotion; however, the chapter on "Financial Considerations" (pp. 28–35) includes an excellent basic and practical discussion of the costs involved in online search services; costing, including subsidized use of online services and full cost versus partial cost recovery; and charging for online services using a fixed price versus a per minute pricing algorithm. "It is strongly suggested that the service not be totally free to the user" to avoid "frivolous" use of the system. Advice for billing the patron is given, along with information about vendor bills.

COST ANALYSIS

Bement, James H. "The New Prices—Some Comparisons." *Online* 1 (April 1977): 9–22.

The costs of using BRS, SDC and DIALOG are compared. While the price schedules are outdated, methodology for comparison remains relevant.

Boyce, Bert R. "A Cost Accounting Model for Online Computerized Literature Searching." *Journal of Library Administration* 4 (Summer 1983):43–9.

The discussion of cost accounting in the library literature is "sparse." A model for costing online services is presented that accounts for direct (variable and fixed) costs and indirect fixed costs. The "sum of the direct variable costs plus the direct fixed cost increment" equals the search costs.

Boyce, Bert R., and Gillen, Edward J. "Is It More Cost-Effective to Print On- or Offline?" *RQ* 21 (Winter 1981):117–20.

Using a formula to determine when local print cost per citation is more cost-effective, the authors apply it to searching AGRICOLA, ERIC and NTIS on SDC or DIALOG. Dependent on length of citation, terminal speed and citation charges, online printing was more cost-effective.

Buntrock, Robert E. "Cost Effectiveness of On-Line Searching of Chemical Information: An Industrial Viewpoint." *Journal of Chemical Information and Computer Science* 24 (May
1984):54–7.

The article reviews cost-effectiveness of online searching
including online versus manual searching, vendor comparisons, searcher experience as a productivity variable, etc. The
overall viewpoint is on chemical information.

Cable, Leslie G. "Cost Analysis of Reference Service to Outside Users." *Bulletin of the Medical Library Association* 68
(April 1980):247–8.

A cost analysis of staff time required to provide reference
service to outside users at the University of Oregon Health
Sciences Center Libraries resulted in an estimate of $5.18 per
search.

Calkins, Mary L. "On-Line Services and Operational Costs."
Special Libraries 68 (January 1977):13–7.

A cost study of online searches performed at the Environmental Protection Agency's Cincinnati library via DIALOG,
SDC, MEDLINE, and TOXLINE, revealed "the cost-effectiveness of on-line literature searching as compared with manual and batch searching." Online searches averaged $25.31
per search, versus $150 for manual and $350 for batch
searches.

Cooper, Michael D., and Dewath, Nancy A. "The Cost of
On-Line Bibliographic Searching." *Journal of Library Automation* 9 (September 1976):195–209.

A cost analysis of online searching at four public libraries
using DIALOG revealed an average of $28.41 (excluding
phone line charges) per search. Costs included database
charges, offline charges, and labor. There was wide variation
among libraries and searchers in the time required to perform
searches.

Cooper, Michael D., and DeWath, Nancy A. "The Effect of
User Fees on the Cost of On-Line Searching in Libraries."
Journal of Library Automation 10 (December 1977):304–19.

This is a highly research-oriented article which compares

the cost and time of providing online search services in a group of public libraries. The analysis was confined to search costs (staff and database charges) and did not approach cost-effectiveness of online searching. The primary finding was that when the library charged a fee, the staff took more time to prepare and follow up on the search, and spent less time online, thus reducing vendor costs. This effectively shifted a proportion of the search costs from the patron, who paid for certain vendor expenses, to the library, which paid for the staff time. Costs to the library averaged $26.73 when the search was free, and $28.78 when a fee was charged. The cost analysis involved searching via DIALOG.

Cornell, Joseph A. et al. "Cost Comparison of Searching the Iowa Drug Information Service Index Manually and by Computer." *American Journal of Hospital Pharmacy* 38 (May 1981):680–4.

A study of the costs of using the Iowa Drug Information Services Index manually and by computer found that the computer system was less expensive. Costs analyzed included start-up and maintenance costs.

Divilbiss, J.L., and Self, Phyllis C. "Work Analysis by Random Sampling." *Bulletin of the Medical Library Association* 66 (January 1978):19–23.

Random sampling by using an electronic alarm device provided a means to analyze work activities. Using such a technique to determine percentages of staff time for each activity provides, among other management data, the basis for cost allocations.

Drake, Miriam A. "Attribution of Library Costs." *College & Research Libraries* 38 (November 1977):514–9.

Cost studies in four academic libraries are summarized. Cost allocation methods include dividing costs according to faculty size, distributing indirect costs based on faculty salaries, and allocating by library use. A cost study performed at the Purdue University Libraries is presented.

Drinan, Helen. "Financial Management of Online Services— A How-to Guide." *Online* 3 (October 1979):14–21.

The author presents a model for "cost-recovery based financial management of online services in any information center." The method is based on break-even analysis, balancing expenses against user charges. The model covers three financial tasks—budgeting, pricing, and controlling. Budgeting includes monitoring demand from past experience and compiling a cost item inventory of direct labor, direct expenses and indirect expenses. Fixed versus variable costs are discussed in relation to direct and indirect expenses. Pricing is a method of analyzing the budget to determine rational cost allocation. Costing can be for full costing (includes direct and indirect costs) or direct costing (only direct costs). The method for determining direct costing is illustrated, followed by the methods for allocating indirect expenses using either a flat service fee or a surcharge. Controlling costs completes the financial management process through a formal year-end reporting system. Whether or not fees are actually charged, this financial model assists in cost management.

Elchesen, Dennis R. "Cost-Effectiveness Comparison of Manual and Online Retrospective Bibliographic Searching." *Journal of the American Society for Information Science* 29 (March 1978):56–66.

This comparison concludes, as so many earlier studies have, that online searching is less expensive, faster and more effective than manual searching. SDC was used as the search vendor. An appendix provides detailed cost calculations, useful for those interested in methodology.

Elman, Stanley A. "Cost Comparisons of Manual and On-Line Computerized Literature Searching." *Special Libraries* 66 (January 1975):12–8.

This study compares the cost of manual searching with online searching. A formula which captures all cost factors was used; the formula included line time, offline prints, labor, communications, and equipment costs. Online searching was performed on DIALOG, and was considerably less expensive (about one-fifth the cost) than manual searching.

Flynn, T.; Holohan, P.A.; Magson, M.S.; and Munro, J.D. "Cost Effectiveness Comparison of Online and Manual Bibliographic Information Retrieval." *Journal of Information Science* 1 (May 1979):77–84.

Librarians at ICI, a British-based group of companies, evaluated the cost-effectiveness of manual versus online bibliographic information retrieval. A cost model was developed for use in other libraries. In addition to having a variety of qualitative advantages over manual searching, online searching was shown to be quantitatively more advantageous.

Herstand, Jo Ellen. "Interlibrary Loan Cost Study and Comparison." *RQ* 20 (Spring 1981):249–56.

Interlibrary loan transactions (borrowing and lending) at the University of Oklahoma were collected for a two-week period. Data for the study were analyzed so as to be comparable with the Palmour study on interlibrary loan costs, published in 1972. The method utilized at OU uses a simple formula, can be manually collected, and provides sound, estimated data.

Jensen, Rebecca J.; Asbury, Herbert O.; and King, Radford G. "Costs and Benefits to Industry of Online Literature Searches." *Special Libraries* 71 (July 1980):291–9.

A client survey was conducted that examined user-identified dollar costs and benefits of an online literature search. The results showed a direct relationship (a ratio of 2.9 to 1) between client dollars invested and benefits derived from the search. The user's perception of costs and benefits is necessary to the evaluation of information systems. Libraries tend to think only in terms of direct costs for providing the search rather than costs borne by the user such as the user's presearch time.

Kantor, Paul B. "Cost and Usage of Health Sciences Libraries: Economic Aspects." *Bulletin of the Medical Library Association* 72 (July 1984):274–86.

In a research study of ninety-five health sciences libraries located in three geographic areas, costs and use of three principle services—circulation of materials, reference services and inhouse use of materials—were analyzed. Results are presented as total national costs by type of library and by user type versus purpose of use (patient care, research, education, and other). Costs by user type, average unit cost of services and allocation of overhead are among the other results presented.

Kaya, Birsen, and Hurlebaus, Alice. "Comparison of United Parcel Service and United States Postal Service Delivery Speed and Cost for Interlibrary Loan." *Bulletin of the Medical Library Association* 66 (July 1978):345–6.

The article discusses both speed and cost of delivery of ILL using two different delivery methods. Cost analysis is quite limited.

Keller, John E. "Program Budgeting and Cost Benefit Analysis in Libraries." *College & Research Libraries* 30 (March 1969):156–60.

The author advocates program budgeting and cost benefit analysis for use in academic libraries. Despite its publication date (1969), the article is included here because of the importance of these concepts for managerial decision making in libraries.

King, Donald W. "Pricing Policies in Academic Libraries." *Library Trends* 28 (Summer 1979):47–62.

King discusses pricing in economic terms, e.g., using the cost and quantity demanded and price and quantity demanded relationships. Journal use and interlibrary loan are used as examples. This is part of a thematic issue on "The Economics of Academic Libraries."

Koch, Jean E. "A Review of the Costs and Cost-Effectiveness of Online Bibliographic Searching." *Reference Services Review* 10 (January–March 1982):59–64.

Costs and cost analysis of online bibliographic searching are briefly reviewed. Online costs are discussed in terms of support costs, production costs, and overhead; other topics include a comparison of manual versus online searching and pricing alternatives.

Lopez, Manuel D. "Academic Reference Service: Measurement, Costs and Value." *RQ* 12 (Spring 1973):234–42.

Methods and rationale for measuring reference services, in particular reference information questions, are reviewed. Cost analysis may have been avoided by reference librarians because they "do not want to know the cost of their present operations and are intimidated by cost accounting systems"; cost analysis is a powerful budgeting tool. Measurement of services, to be meaningful, must be evaluated against criteria or standards.

Lutz, Raymond P. "Costing Information Centers." *Bulletin of the Medical Library Association* 59 (April 1971):254–61.

Information services provided to nonprimary clientele are frequently based on cost recovery. This article discusses the basis for establishing user charges; cost analysis based on full cost pricing, total unit cost pricing, and value added pricing; and implementation of a cost analysis system which is dependent on predicting and achieving a level of service request volume and types of services to be offered.

Martyn, John, and Lancaster, F. Wilfrid. *Investigative Methods in Library and Information Science: An Introduction.* Chapter 4. "Cost Analysis." Arlington, Va.: Information Resources Press, 1981, pp. 175–92.

The book as a whole discusses methods for analyzing and evaluating information services. Cost analysis is one measure of effectiveness. The British Prestel System is analyzed as an example of costing. Cost-effectiveness and cost-benefit analyses are discussed.

Mitchell, Betty Jo; Tanis, Norman E.; and Jaffe, Jack. *Cost Analysis of Library Functions; A Total System Approach.* Greenwich, Connecticut: Jai Press, 1978.

The cost accounting system of California State University, Northridge (CSUN) library is used as a model for other libraries to make decisions. Cost accounting should be a continuous management tool for daily operations. The model used at CSUN is a detailed computer program based on production units, activities or tasks, and organizational units.

Saffady, William. "The Economics of Online Bibliographic Searching: Costs and Cost Justifications." *Library Technology Reports* 15 (September–October 1979):567–653.

This report "examines the costs associated with, and the potential for cost justification inherent in, the library use of online bibliographic search services." Although actual costs and figures would now be outdated, the methodology presented in this article for calculating costs and analyzing cost justification remains useful.

Schneiweiss, Fred. "Use and Cost Analysis of Online Literature Searching in a University-Based Drug Information Center." *American Journal of Hospital Pharmacy* 40 (February 1983):254–6.

The use of online literature searching in a drug information center over a three-year period is described. MEDLINE was the predominant database. Cost analysis is limited to vendor (BRS) charges including contract, royalties, telecommunications, and offline prints.

Shirley, Sherrilynne. "A Survey of Computer Search Service Costs in the Academic Health Sciences Library." *Bulletin of the Medical Library Association* 66 (October 1978):390–6.

A very lucid and practical approach to cost analysis, this article surveys in detail the "costs involved in the provision of computer search services beyond vendor charges for connect time and printing." The analysis, conducted at the Norris Medical Library, University of Southern California, discusses online search services in terms of production costs, consisting primarily of direct online search costs and personnel time; support costs, which are divided into start-up and recurring costs; and overhead costs. Methods for price setting, such as a unit charge per search (fixed rate) and a variable rate, are discussed. Appendices give a method for calculating a fixed rate search charge and a detailed cost analysis for online searches.

Spencer, Carol C. "Random Time Sampling With Self-Observation for Library Cost Studies: Unit Costs of Interlibrary Loans and Photocopies at a Regional Medical Library." *Journal of the American Society for Information Science* 22 (May–June 1971):153–60.

This research article uses random time sampling to determine labor costs for providing interlibrary loan and photocopy service at the Mid-Eastern Regional Medical Library, College of Physicians of Philadelphia. Labor costs, added to other known costs (such as materials, equipment and overhead) resulted in a unit cost per request of $1.526 for loans and $1.534 for photocopies. Thus, "the cost of providing a photocopy did not exceed the cost of lending an original document." While the unit costs may be dated, the methodology for determining the labor costs remains valid.

Spencer, Carol C. "Random Time Sampling with Self-Observation for Library Cost Studies: Unit Costs of Reference Questions." *Bulletin of the Medical Library Association* 68 (January 1980):53–7.

Random alarm devices, plus a checklist of categories of reference questions, were used to determine unit costs of reference questions at the National Library of Medicine. Percentage of time spent on each category of question was translated into unit costs; representative wage costs were $.44 for directional questions, $1.98 for quick reference and $4.57 for extended reference.

Spencer, Carol C. "Unit Costs of Interlibrary Loans and Photocopies at a Regional Medical Library: Preliminary Report." *Bulletin of the Medical Library Association* 58 (April 1970):189–90.

The unit costs of providing interlibrary loans and photocopies at the Mid-Eastern Regional Medical Library were $1.932 for originals and $1.763 for photocopies. While the costs are outdated the method used (Random Alarm Mechanisms) deserves further attention.

Wish, John; Collins, Craig; and Jacobson, Vance. "Terminal Costs for On-line Searching." *College & Research Libraries* 38 (July 1977):291–7.

Cost analysis is used to determine the most cost-effective terminal for online searching. Variable costs, primarily the number of searches performed per month, takes precedence over fixed costs in choosing a terminal.

Zais, Harriet W. "Economic Modeling: An Aid to the Pricing of Information Services." *Journal of the American Society for Information Science* 28 (March 1977):89–95.

This article is an excellent place for librarians to become

accustomed to the terminology and techniques of pricing practices. The article defines and discusses such concepts as: cost-based pricing, demand-based pricing, competition-based pricing, fixed costs, variable costs, marginal cost, average-cost pricing, price elasticity of demand, price discrimination and marginal cost pricing. The author views pricing as an art. Throughout the article, pricing of SDI services is used as an example.

COST RECOVERY

Arcari, Ralph D. "Clinical Librarian Program—Cost Recovery Effort." *Clinical Librarian Quarterly* 1 (December 1982):-7–10.

The clinical librarian program of the University of Connecticut Health Center Library finances its services from the departments involved through a cost recovery effort.

Brantz, Malcolm H. "State-wide Cost Recovery for Health Science Audiovisual Loan Service in Connecticut." *Bulletin of the Medical Library Association* 72 (July 1984):266–9.

The University of Connecticut Health Center Library's successful statewide cost recovery AV service for nurses was originally funded by a federal grant but is now operated on a fee-for-service basis. With the imposition of fees (unspecified), average loans per week dropped from one hundred to fifteen, but are gradually increasing. AV equipment is rented within the state at a cost recovery rate ($65.00).

Heinlen, William F., and Midbon, Mark A. "Data Base Management on a Budget." *RQ* 18 (Fall 1978):50–2.

Management aspects of initiating online searching in a library with limited resources are described. In addition to determining costs (e.g., training, direct costs, etc.), cost recovery through fee for direct costs was necessary.

Kenton, David. "The Development of a More Equitable Method of Billing for Online Services." *Online* 8 (September 1984):13–7.

The National Library of Medicine has developed a new and

innovative method of billing for MEDLINE use based upon the work performed and data delivered as opposed to connect hours. The rationale behind the change, implemented October 1, 1983, is presented along with a discussion of the new algorithm. Criteria for implementation of the new structure are listed.

Lyders, Richard; Eckels, Diane; and Leatherbury, Maurice C. "Cost Allocation and Cost Generation." In: *New Horizons for Academic Libraries,* edited by Robert D. Stueart and Richard D. Johnson. New York: K.G. Saur Publishing, Inc., 1979, pp. 116–22.

A three factor method for budget allocation is used by the Houston Academy of Medicine—Texas Medical Center Library, based on an assessment to each user institution, the size of facilities and student bodies of each institution, and use of the library by each institution's faculty, staff and students.

Rousmaniere, Peter F.; Ciarkowski, Elaine F.; and Guild, Nathaniel. "Bridging the Library Budget Gap; An Approach to Creating Fair User Charges." *College & Research Libraries News* 44 (March 1983):69–71.

The Countway Library of Medicine at Harvard Medical School, with the aid of a consulting firm, designed a user charge system that was based on two databases. The cost database was built on nineteen services which were allocated to seventeen cost centers, while the user database was developed from three week-long surveys. The study required "a careful cost analysis and user survey effort." Costs for library services were passed on to affiliated institutions based on a "schedule of assessments."

Schultz, Claire K. "Establishing Cost Centers Within Libraries of Medical Centers." *Bulletin of the Medical Library Association* 71 (January 1983):1–5.

Schultz advocates running medical center libraries in a businesslike manner to analyze and recover costs. The methodology used for analysis is the establishment of cost centers within the library, in which library costs are divided into public, technical and administrative services, which then can be charged back to teaching, patient care, or research.

MARKETING

Andreasen, Alan R. "Advancing Library Marketing." *Journal of Library Administration* 1 (Fall 1980):17–32.

Marketing has been enthusiastically accepted by libraries. Areas for improving the applications are: correction of misapplications, e.g., confusing selling with marketing; upgrading present applications, e.g., using multivariate analysis and segmentation techniques; and introducing new applications, e.g., using innovative management principles such as brainstorming, critical path planning, forecasting, test marketing, and focus groups.

Andreasen, Alan R. "Nonprofits: Check Your Attention to Customers." *Harvard Business Review* 60 (May–June 1982): 105–10.

The author feels that not enough attention is focused on clients, and that nonprofit organizations should be more customer than product-oriented.

Baker, Michael J., ed. *Marketing in Adversity.* New York: MacMillan Press, 1976.

Marketing in non-traditional situations is the theme of this British-based book. Especially relevant to libraries are the chapters on "The Consumer, The Market Place and the Marketing Mix," and "Marketing: Not for Profit."

Bellardo, Trudi, and Waldhart, Thomas J. "Marketing Products and Services in Academic Libraries." *Libri* 27 (September 1977):181–94.

In this excellent overview, marketing is discussed in the context of academic libraries. Both market analysis and the marketing mix are extensively analyzed, with an emphasis on the fact that libraries generally are marketing services as opposed to products, and that libraries have two separate "publics": the sources for funding and the library clients. A fairly extensive treatment of fees for online search services is presented in the "price" section of the marketing mix.

Berry, John. "The 'Marketization' of Libraries." *Library Journal* 106 (January 1, 1981):5.

Berry debates the need for marketing library services,

where a dependence for a product is created, versus building an individual's self-reliance for finding information.

Berry, Leonard L. "Services Marketing is Different." *Business* 30 (May/June 1980):24–9.
Relative intangibility, lack of standardization, and simultaneous production and consumption of services makes marketing services different from other goods. Some of the important tools for marketing services are: customizing service, appearance of the service provider, and reshaping demand.

Carroll, Daniel. "Library Marketing: Old and New Truths." *Wilson Library Bulletin* 57 (November 1982):212–6.
Libraries and other not-for-profit institutions have always been engaged in "passive marketing." Contained here are ten "old truths" and "new truths" which present marketing for libraries as being active and protagonistic.

Crane, Nancy B., and Pilachowski, David M. "Introducing Online Bibliographic Service to its Users: The Online Presentation." *Online* 2 (October 1978):20–9.
Crane and Pilachowski focus on one specific aspect of the marketing process: promotion. In this case, they give hints on introducing online service to new users. A list of advantages and disadvantages helps the searcher anticipate questions from the audience, while a list of "do's" and "don'ts" gives some useful tips.

Cronin, Blaise. "New Technology and Marketing—the Challenge for Librarians." *Aslib Proceedings* 34 (September 1982):377–93.
Primary aspects of marketing are communication and exchange. Information needs, analysis and market segmentation are important in the marketing of services. Throughout the article, health science professionals provide examples of library users; computerization provides the example of the service.

Donnelley, James H., and George, William R. *Marketing of Services.* Chicago, Illinois: American Marketing Association, 1981.
The result of the first AMA conference focusing solely on

marketing service, this collection of papers covers a wide range of marketing strategies in commercial, professional and nonprofit/public sector services.

Dragon, Andrea. "Marketing and the Public Library." *Public Library Quarterly* 4 (Winter 1983):37–46.

This is the first in a series of articles on marketing in public libraries. The primary focus is the library's product, including product strategy, new product development, the product life cycle, and why products fail. Libraries should develop a product strategy that appeals to various market segments that have been targeted by the library.

Dragon, Andrea C. "Marketing Communications for Libraries." *Public Library Quarterly* 5 (Spring 1984):63–77.

This is the second in a series of articles on marketing. While the examples are from public libraries, the discussion of the role of communication is applicable to all libraries. The library must be able to identify the target audience and the target market for a message. Designing promotional messages is discussed, and advertising, public relations, and publicity are defined and differentiated. The author notes that volunteers are public relations agents.

Dragon, Andrea C. "Marketing the Library." *Wilson Library Bulletin* 53 (March 1979):498–502.

This article provides valuable, practical advice on marketing techniques. The author lays a firm foundation on the need for and value of marketing, and gives specific examples for utilizing the traditional mechanisms of price, product, promotion, and place in the public library situation. The techniques and rationales are easily transferable to special, medical and academic libraries.

Dunn, Ronald G., and Boyle, Harry F. "On-Line Searching: Costly or Cost Effective? A Marketing Perspective." *Journal of Chemical Information & Computer Science* 24 (May 1984):51–4.

Too much emphasis has been placed on analyzing the actual or direct costs of online searching. Value as perceived by the customer is different from the price of acquiring information, since there are many other "costs" than the evident or measurable costs. A marketing approach would educate the customer as to the value of information.

Edinger, Joyce A. "Marketing Library Services: Strategy for Survival." *College & Research Libraries* 41 (July 1980):328–32.

Marketing "refers to the effective management by an organization of its exchange relations with its various publics," and is as applicable to libraries and other nonprofit organizations as it is to profit making organizations. For successful implementation of a marketing program, libraries must have a top down commitment to the marketing concept (i.e., a user orientatation), and a systematic marketing audit, requiring an organized approach, is recommended. The four factors of the marketing mix (product, place, price, and promotion) are discussed in terms of library services and programs. The article concludes by asking the question, "How can libraries afford *not* to market their services?"

Elias, A. "Marketing for Online Bibliographic Services." *Online Review* 3 (1979):107–17.

Marketing online services is discussed from the database producer's viewpoint, in particular, BIOSIS Previews. A fundamental question is whether "we are marketing a product or a service." A multi-directional market model is presented, along with data for various market segments.

Emerging Perspectives on Services Marketing, edited by Leonard L. Berry, G. Lynn Shostack, and Gregory D. Upah. Chicago, Ill.: American Marketing Association, 1983. (Proceedings Series/American Marketing Association.)

This proceedings covers a variety of aspects of marketing services from consumer satisfaction and evaluation, innovation, and issues in new service development, to implementing services marketing, research priorities, and design of services.

Ferguson, Douglas. "Marketing Online Services in the University." *Online* 1 (July 1977):15–23.

Marketing of online services is presented from a very practical perspective. Above all, marketing is user-oriented—the consumer's needs must be placed first. Examples are given for publicity, management issues are presented, and pricing is discussed as part of marketing.

Freeman, James E., and Katz, Ruth M. "Information Marketing." In: *Annual Review of Information Science,* V.13, edited by Martha E. Williams. Washington, D.C.: American Society for Information Science, 1978, pp. 37–59.

This is a review of the literature on information marketing. Discussed also are: pricing, fees for service and information brokers.

Goldstucker, Jac L., ed., and Goodwin, Dennis W., comp. *Marketing Information: A Professional Reference Guide.* Atlanta, Ga.: College of Business Administration, Georgia State University, 1982.

This is an outstanding guide to the literature and sources for marketing information. The first section lists associations and organizations, including special libraries, research centers, continuing education programs, and government agencies. The second section is an annotated list of sources of marketing information, divided first by general subject (e.g., advertising, pricing, public relations and sales forecasting), and within each subject by books, periodicals, AV materials (if available) and databases (if available). Title and publisher indexes aid in finding information.

Graef, Jean L., and Greenwood, Larry. "Marketing Library Services: A Case Study in Providing Bibliographic Instruction in an Academic Library." In: *New Horizons for Academic Libraries,* edited by Robert D. Stueart and Richard D. Johnson. New York: K.G. Saur Publishing Inc., 1979, pp. 212–28.

The University of Kentucky library initiated bibliographic instruction by creating a marketing program that used a "marketing mix" of price, product, promotion, personal selling and distribution.

Gwynn, M. Beth. "Marketing the Law School Library." *Law Library Journal* 71 (May 1978):234–46.

The implementation of a marketing orientation in a law

school library is described. The concepts of customer satisfaction, exchange, organizational responsiveness and the intelligent consumer are applicable in all types of libraries.

Keeler, Elizabeth. "Mainstreaming the New Library." *Special Libraries* 73 (October 1982):260–5.

An approach of marketing, production, and advertising is suggested to move the library from the traditional role of warehouse into "true information management." Of necessity, this involves the library in the political realities of the institution. Marketing and advertising are ways to make the library's services or products indispensable to the organization.

Klement, Susan. "Marketing Library-Related Expertise." *Canadian Library Journal* 34 (April 1977):97–101.

The article discusses a special project by the Metropolitan Toronto Library, in which a list of consultants, mostly librarians, was developed to fill a local need for referral and consultation help.

Kotler, Philip. *Marketing for Nonprofit Organizations.* 2nd edition. Englewood Cliffs, N.J.: Prentice Hall, 1982.

Kotler is *the classic* for marketing in nonprofit organizations. This second edition updates the 1975 edition. Primary sections in the book are: Understanding Marketing (includes strategic planning); Organizing Marketing; Analyzing Marketing Opportunities (includes forecasting, segmentation, targeting, and consumer analysis); Planning the Marketing Mix (includes programming, budgeting, price decisions, advertising, promotion, and public relations); Attracting Resources; and Adapting Marketing.

Kotler, Philip. "Strategic Planning and the Marketing Process." *Business* 30 (May/June 1980):2–9.

The performance of a business or organization is dependent on its creative alignment with the environment. Strategic planning develops and maintains a strategic fit with the environment while marketing seeks to identify and analyze opportunities "to fulfill the company's mission and objectives." Principles stated in this article can be translated for use by libraries.

Kotler, Philip. "Strategies for Introducing Marketing into Nonprofit Organizations." *Journal of Marketing* 43 (January 1979): 37–44.

Nonprofits (e.g., universities and hospitals) are becoming interested in marketing. To implement a successful marketing program, Kotler recommends that the institution appoint a marketing committee and task forces, consider a marketing consultant to carry out a marketing audit, and eventually appoint a marketing director or marketing vice president.

Kranich, Nancy. "Fees for Library Service: They are not Inevitable!" *Library Journal* 105 (May 1, 1980):1048–51.

Written from the public library perspective, this article focuses on concepts such as equal access to library services (considered public goods), the economics of financing services (e.g., financing should be diversified), and priorities for services. In the long run, the author concludes, fees are not inevitable.

Levitt, Theodore. "Marketing Intangible Products and Product Intangibles." *Harvard Business Review* 81 (May/June 1981):94–102.

Rather than speaking of services and goods, intangibles and tangibles may be a better distinction. All products have some type of intangible aspects. With intangible products (primarily services), the "customers usually don't know what they're getting until they don't get it." People usually voice only dissatisfaction and are not vocal about satisfaction.

Lovelock, Christopher H., and Weinberg, Charles B. "Public and Nonprofit Marketing Comes of Age." In: *Review of Marketing 1978,* edited by Gerald Zaltman and Thomas V. Bonoma. Chicago, Il.: American Marketing Association, 1978, pp. 413–52.

Marketing in the public sector is differentiated from nonprofit marketing in that there are several publics, the objective is not profit, services rather than goods are marketed, and there are not market pressures. Also discussed are marketing in health care and in higher education.

Massey, Morris E. "Market Analysis and Audience Research for Libraries." *Library Trends* 24 (January 1976): 473–81.

Massey concentrates his comments on market segmentation, including benefit segmentation, and market research methodologies appropriate for libraries.

Montana, Patrick J., ed. *Marketing in Nonprofit Organizations.* New York: AMACOM, 1978.

A collection of articles (many reprinted from sources such as the *Harvard Business Review* and the *Journal of Marketing*), this book provides practical advice on marketing services in not-for-profit organizations. A matrix at the front of the book indicates which articles are relevant to the following nonprofit sectors: government, education, health, religious and charitable organizations, and associations. Articles range from basic concepts of marketing by authors such as Kotler and Levy, to lighter, "salesmanship" articles. One particularly good article by Berry and George discusses opportunities for marketing the university in the 1970s, an "era of crisis."

Moulton, Bethe, "Marketing and Library Cooperatives." *Wilson Library Bulletin* 55 (January 1981):347–52.

Marketing begins with a recognition that organizations are involved in an exchange process with individuals or other organizations. As service organizations, it is appropriate that libraries use marketing to plan for service delivery. Marketing analysis, customer analysis, organizational analysis, competitive analysis, defining one's business, and the marketing mix (product, price, place, and promotion) are presented as tools for organizing a marketing approach for library cooperatives. Interestingly, while the article's focus is on networking, the introduction of MEDLINE to hospital library users is utilized as an example of customer analysis and promotion of a new service.

Oldman, Christine, "Marketing Library and Information Services." *European Journal of Marketing* 11 (1977):460–74.

Information services are discussed in this article in terms of the consumer behavior side of marketing. The author also presents the concept of "information need."

Olsen, James L., Jr. "Unlocking the Library's Market—Seven Keys." In: *Special Librarianship: A New Reader,* by Eugene B. Jackson. Metuchen, N.J.: Scarecrow Press, 1980, pp. 449–56.
Personal experience provides the basis for Olsen's tips on marketing. Among the seven keys are knowing your organizational structure and the people, communicating with management, and innovation.

Rados, David L. *Marketing for Non-Profit Organizations.* Boston, Ma.: Auburn House, 1981.
This text is "about the marketing problems that arise in non-profit organizations." Discussed are costs, behavior (segmentation, marketing research), marketing strategy, distribution, communications, price, and marketing control and marketing organization. Case studies are included for classroom use.

Radway, Gerry, and Steward, Connie. "Promoting Online Literature Searching." In: *Library Management in Review,* edited by A. Bruemmer et al., New York: Special Libraries Association, 1981.
A variety of techniques for promoting online searching at the G.E. Electronics Park Library are described. The article includes a list of "Tips for Promoting Online Services."

Schmidt, Janet A. "How to Promote Online Services to the People Who Count the Most . . . Management . . . End Users." *Online* 1 (January 1977):32–8.
Tips for justifying online services to management are suggested, along with promotional ideas. The primary promotional tool is the online demonstration; tips include an online reception and special group presentations.

Schmidt, Janet. "Outline for an Online Public Relations Program." *Online* 2 (October 1978):47–50.
Public relations is one aspect of marketing. The information in this article is designed to make online searching more visible within the institution.

Schwartz, Diane G. "Bibliographic Instruction: A Public Relations Perspective." *Medical Reference Services Quarterly* 3 (Summer 1984):43–9.

Public relations is one aspect of marketing. Three phases for a public relations program for bibliographic instruction are given: market audit, communication, and promotion.

Sciandra, Russell C., and Stein, Judith A. "Applying Marketing Techniques to Promotion of the Cancer Information Service." *Progress in Clinical and Biological Research* 130 (1983):153–60.

A Task Force from the Cancer Information Service applied "social marketing techniques to the development of a comprehensive promotion plan." "Social marketing" involves applying marketing to the promotion of socially beneficial causes. Marketing research was conducted to assess the needs, views and characteristics of the audience; the audience was segmented; and plans were developed to target individual segments. Outreach programs should be based "on sound research into the cancer-related knowledge, attitudes and practices of a diverse populace."

Shapiro, Benson P. "Marketing for Nonprofit Organizations." *Harvard Business Review* 51 (September 1973):123–32.

This contribution from the business literature discusses marketing for nonprofit organizations based on the author's experience. After identifying the three major marketing tasks of the nonprofit manager (resource attraction, resource allocation, and persuasion), he describes the marketing mix (communication, distribution, pricing, and product).

Shapiro, Stanley J. "Marketing and the Information Professional: Odd Couple or Meaningful Relationship?" *Special Libraries* 71 (November 1980):469–74.

Marketing is presented as "an attitude, an approach, and a set of relevant tools, techniques, and concepts." The attitude is positive and responsive; the approach segments the market, matches services to users, and develops a systematic marketing plan; and the set of tools, techniques and concepts utilize the four P's (product, price, promotion, and place) to develop and implement the marketing plan. The concept of the librarian as a corporate information manager is presented along with the need for joint MLS-MBA programs.

Shostack, G. Lynn. "The Service Marketing Frontier." In: *Review of Marketing 1978,* edited by Gerald Zaltman and Thomas V. Bonoma. Chicago, Il.: American Marketing Association, 1978, pp. 373–88.

This overview of services marketing discusses the characteristics in a service environment, service distribution, service levels and differentiation, and the "human factor" in service marketing.

Smith, Patricia K. "Marketing Online Services." *Online* 4 (January 1980): 60–2; Part 2, *Online* 4 (April 1980): 68–9.

This is a basic introduction to the marketing of online services. The rationale behind a marketing strategy, segmentation, promotion and selling services, product design, and pricing are all discussed. Online services can be considered a specialty good.

Smith, Roy. "And the Library Entrepreneur." *Canadian Library Journal* 40 (October 1983):263–6.

Sutton, England's public library generates about twenty-five percent of its operating budget from a variety of innovative ideas. Using razzmatazz, showmanship and a variety of unique activities, the library makes its presence known in the community. Although the article is still in "speech" format, the marketing ideas are creative and stir the imagination.

Southern Marketing Association. *Progress in Marketing Theory and Practice,* edited by Ronald D. Taylor, John H. Summey, and Blaise J. Bergiel. Carbondale, Il.: Southern Marketing Association, 1981.

The papers in this volume were presented at the annual meeting of the Southern Marketing Association. Relevant papers on nonprofits, services or university marketing are by Davis and Joyce (pp. 25–8); Cooper, Reidenbach and Sherrell (pp. 228–31); and Madden and Walter (pp. 311–5).

Sterngold, Arthur. "Marketing for Special Libraries and Information Centers: The Positioning Process." *Special Libraries* 73 (October 1982):254–8.

Internal marketing is presented as an essential function of information management. The library or information center must position itself to effectively operate and meet the needs of its clientele. The two keys are focusing the marketing program on specific groups of users and concentrating on which information needs will be served. A library which repositions itself to meet the changing needs of its institution is used to illustrate the need to be aware of institutional goals, objectives and priorities.

Thomas, Dan R.E. "Strategy is Different in Service Business." *Harvard Business Review* 78 (July/August 1978):158–65.

Service businesses have unique opportunities to build barriers to entry (ex.: economies of scale, proprietary technology and service differentiation), for cutting costs, and for competing price. A comment on price competition is that setting a price too low is as problematic as setting it too high.

Weinstock, M. "Marketing Scientific and Technical Information Service." In: *Encyclopedia of Library and Information Science,* edited by Allen Kent. Volume 17. New York: Marcel Dekker, 1976, pp. 165–88.

This overview of marketing gives basic information on such topics as market analysis and segmentation, new product planning, and market planning and implementation. Sales forecasting, marketing strategies, promotion and pricing also are discussed.

Wood, Elizabeth J. "Strategic Planning and the Marketing Process: Library Applications." *Journal of Academic Librarianship* 9 (March 1983):15–20.

The business concepts of marketing and strategic planning are explored in relation to library applications. Strategic planning is characterized as the process of fitting the organization's basic mission with its market opportunities. Awareness of the environment and building on the strengths of the organizations are essential. Marketing is presented in four steps: marketing opportunity analysis, target market selection, marketing mix strategy, and marketing systems development.

Yorke, D.A. *Marketing the Library Service.* London: Library Association, 1977. (Library Association Management Pamphlets, #3).

This fifty-one page pamphlet, published by the (British) Library Association, looks at marketing as a philosophy, discussing its role, marketing characteristics and research techniques, demand, and the product/service life cycle. Positioning of the library, both academic and public, is discussed, along with a plan of marketing action.

FEE-FOR-SERVICE

Association of Research Libraries. Office of Management Studies. *Fees for Services.* Washington, D.C.: Association of Research Libaries, 1981. (Systems & Procedure Exchange Center SPEC Kit #74).

This SPEC kit contains material produced by libraries already charging fees that will aid libraries intending to establish fee-based services. Included are policies on general fees for service, an evaluation of the effect of fees on borrowing, documents for photocopy services, documents for ILL policy and online search services, and examples of public services policy publicity.

Beeler, Richard J., and Lueck, Antoinette L. "Pricing of Online Services for Nonprimary Clientele." *Journal of Academic Librarianship* 10 (May 1984):69–72.

A survey of 133 university libraries revealed that between eighty and ninety percent made online services available to off-campus, or nonprimary, clientele; of those offering service to off-campus users, almost seventy percent charged a different rate (higher) than was charged to students, faculty or staff of their university. Pricing structures for the additional fee (fixed amount, percentage of direct search costs, hourly rate, etc.) are discussed, along with the concept of, and justifications for, price discrimination.

Blake, Fay M., and Perlmutter, Edith L. "The Rush to User Fees: Alternative Proposals." *Library Journal* 102 (October 1, 1977):2005–8.

A philosophical discussion of the fee versus free issue, the article adamantly opposes fees in publicly supported libraries. Fees may cause more problems than might be expected. Alternatives to fees involve tax policy and political priorities.

Blazek, Ron. "User Fees: A Survey of Public and Academic Reference Librarians." *Reference Librarian* 4 (Summer 1982):55–74.

A survey of public and academic (two and four-year colleges) libraries in Florida revealed public reference librarians opposed fees more than academic reference librarians.

Budd, John. "The Terminal and the Terminus: The Prospect of Free Online Bibliographic Searching." *RQ* 21 (Summer 1982):373–8.

The subject of fees for online bibliographic searching is reviewed philosophically, with the conclusion that free online searching is both practically and ideologically feasible and that libraries can budget for free searching.

Burrows, Suzetta, and La Rocco, August. "Fees for Automated Reference Services in Academic Health Science Libraries: No Free Lunches." *Medical Reference Services Quarterly* 2 (Summer 1983):1–11.

Fees for online bibliographic searching are routine in academic health sciences libraries. Philosophical and economic decisions are discussed along with the various bases for fees. The fee structure for online searches at the University of Miami School of Medicine is described in detail.

Cady, Susan A., and Richards, Berry G. "The One-Thousand-Dollar Alternative." *American Libraries* 13 (March 1982):175–6.

The initiation and provision of a fee-based information service for local industry by the Lehigh University Libraries is discussed. Businesses can receive service through a subscription or on a pay-as-you-go basis. Costing, the fee structure and marketing efforts are detailed. Speed of service, confidentiality, and conflict of interest with other library programs also are presented.

Cheshier, Robert G. "Fees for Service in Medical Library Networks." *Bulletin of the Medical Library Association* 60 (April 1972):325–32.

One of the early descriptions of fees for service, this article presents both a philosophical discussion of fees and the role of NLM and resource libraries in document delivery. Also described is the Cleveland Health Sciences Library's fee-for-service arrangement with local libraries, which is based on Institutional Memberships.

Cogswell, James A. "On-Line Search Services: Implications for Libraries and Library Users." *College & Research Libraries* 39 (July 1978):275–80.

Among the major implications for both libraries and library users is the necessity of charging fees to patrons to recover online search costs. The article discusses user attitudes toward fees and overall cost increases of providing online searches.

Conference on Fee Based Research in College and University Libraries. Proceedings of the Meetings at C.W. Post Center of Long Island University, Greenvale, New York, June 17–18, 1982. Greenvale, N.Y.: Center for Business Research, B. Davis Schwartz Memorial Library, C.W. Post Center, Long Island University, c1983.

Based on a conference held at the C.W. Post Center, the proceedings cover all aspects of fee-based research services in academic libraries, including charging, policy considerations, legal considerations and marketing. The prestigious list of authors includes: James Dodd, Miriam Drake, and Mary McNierney Grant.

Cooper, Michael D. "Charging Users for Library Service." *Information Processing and Management* 14 (1978):419–27.

Information possesses both private good and merit good aspects and thus provides a conflict for libraries considering charging a fee for information services. Fee policies for online search services in a public library illustrate the issue. The conclusion is that a certain level or amount of service be supplied free of charge, with direct charges imposed for some users.

Crawford, Paula J., and Thompson, Judith A. "Free Online Searches are Feasible." *Library Journal* 104 (April 1, 1979): 793–5.

At the Library at California State College, Stanislaus, not charging for online searching is considered a necessary prerequisite "if the service is to be treated effectively as an integral part of reference service." The reference librarians utilize professional judgment as to the most effective method of providing the information requested. If a search request is denied, alternative access methods are given to the patron. Free service allows flexibility in that the service will not be limited to those willing and able to pay for online searching. Cost-effectiveness of manual versus online searching is discussed, along with cancellation of the printed counterparts to online databases.

DeGennaro, Richard. "Pay Libraries & User Charges." *Library Journal* 100 (February 15, 1975):363–7.

DeGennaro discusses the history and trends in the issue of fees for library service, suggesting that moderation in views is appropriate. The issue is highly emotional and politically charged, and there is room for a variety of views.

DeWath, Nancy Van House. "Fees for Online Bibliographic Search Services in Publicly-Supported Libraries." *Library Research* 3 (Spring 1981):29–45.

Based on a California Library Association survey of publicly-supported libraries, fees for online search services are discussed in terms of appropriateness of fees, fee structures and implications for future technologies. Over half of the libraries surveyed were public libraries; the remainder were primarily academic libraries. Over forty-three percent did not charge for online searches.

Dodd, James B. "Pay-As-You-Go Plan for Satellite Industrial Libraries Using Academic Facilities." *Special Libraries* 65 (February 1974):66–72.

The development, services, library facilities, and operation of the Georgia Tech Information Exchange Center (IEC) are discussed. The IEC provides services such as photocopying, interlibrary loan, verification, translation, and literature searching for a fee to its clientele. The service is aimed first at the geo-political community comprising the business and industry of Georgia and second to the general (no geographical boundaries) community of science, technology and management. The extensive library holdings and service commitment of the Georgia Tech staff make it cost-effective for outside businesses, even those with corporate libraries, to utilize the IEC.

Dougherty, Richard M. "Editorial: User Fees." *Journal of Academic Librarianship* 3 (January 1978):319.

JAL remains philosophically opposed to user fees. However, if libraries are unable to provide online searching, the private sector, i.e., information brokers, will step in. It is suggested that professional associations should influence public policy to provide funding to libraries so as to prevent the need for user fees.

Drake, Miriam A. "User Fees: A Practical Perspective." Littleton, Colo.: Libraries Unlimited, Inc., 1981.

After a review of the philosophy and issues regarding fees for service in libraries, and a presentation of the opposition views, the book discusses the use of fees in public, academic, and special libraries. Information brokers and their services also are discussed.

Drake, Miriam. "User Fees: Aid or Obstacle to Access?" *Wilson Library Bulletin* 58 (May 1984):632–5.

Using the public library as the focus, Drake discusses the fee versus free question in terms of access to information. After a philosophical approach to the definition of "access," it is pointed out that free service may not actually provide the access to information that is intended. Librarians are reminded that people place value on goods and services by the amount they are willing to pay—implying that free services may be perceived as lacking value.

Ferguson, Douglas. "The Costs of Charging for Information Service." In: *On-Line Bibliographic Services—Where We Are, Where We're Going,* edited by Peter G. Watson. Chicago: American Library Association, Reference and Adult Services Division, April 1977, pp. 60–6.

Four decision areas for determining policies for charging are explored: will there be a charge, who will be charged, what costs will be covered by the charges, and how can an efficient charging system be operated.

Gell, Marilyn Killebrew. "User Fees I: The Economic Argument." *Library Journal* 104 (January 1, 1979):19–23.

This is a purely economic discussion regarding the debate on user fees for library service. Public versus private goods, externalities, and local revenues versus local expenses are presented generically, intentionally avoiding reference to libraries.

Gell, Marilyn Killebrew. "User Fees II: The Library Response." *Library Journal* 104 (January 15, 1979):170–3.

The user fee argument, geared toward public libraries, continues the economic analysis begun in part I. Public libraries are not purely public goods, so that while most services should be offered at a minimum level free of charge, fees should be charged for services which are extraordinary or costly. Public pricing is economically viable and may help the public library preserve basic services.

Huston, Mary M. "Fee or Free: The Effect of Charging on Information Demand." *Library Journal* 104 (September 15, 1979):1811–4.

It is widely accepted that the imposition of fees for online information services reduces the demand for these services. While four studies are cited which provide some insight, this relationship has not been fully studied. Libraries impose fees without fully documenting choice of the fee structure or evaluating the effects of the fees. Equal access to information remains crucial.

Kingman, Nancy M., and Vantine, Carol. "Commentary on the Special Librarian/Fee-Based Service Interface." *Special Libraries* 68 (September 1977):320–22.

Corporations are beginning to realize that, "Information is a resource, just like fuel or other raw materials." INFORM, a fee-based service of the Minneapolis Public Library, is presented as an example of an information service which accesses academic, research and private libraries, as well as other sources, to provide fast, accurate information. The authors emphasize cooperation between librarians and information brokers, and suggest the need for a national network of fee-based services.

Knapp, Sara D. "Beyond Fee or Free." *RQ* 20 (Winter 1980):117–20.

Knapp brings together comments from three libraries which operate "under different systems for charging," and presents descriptions of the systems philosophy or rationales, and results on the effectiveness of the systems. The three libraries are the Pennsylvania State University, which charges direct costs, plus either a fixed $5 fee for internal users or a fifty percent surcharge for external users; California State University, Chico, which operates under a 10-10-10 system where the library and the user share costs; and California State College, Stanislaus, which does not charge for computer searching because of its philosophy of treating online services simply as another reference tool.

Lehman, Lois J., and Wood, M. Sandra. "Effect of Fees on an Information Service for Physicians." *Bulletin of the Medical Library Association* 66 (January 1978): 58–61.

An analysis of an Information Service provided for physicians in Pennsylvania revealed a dramatic decrease in the number of users after fees were implemented.

Linford, John. "To Charge or Not to Charge: A Rationale." *Library Journal* 102 (October 1, 1977):2009–10.

Linford presents a rationale for decision making in regard to fees. Where costs are not incurred or cannot be identified for individual patrons, no charge should be made; however, when costs are incurred for materials which will be used only for an individual patron, a fee should be levied. "Reasonable level of service" is also viable as a guide on whether to charge or not to charge.

Lynch, Mary Jo. *Financing Online Search Services in Publicly Supported Libraries: The Report of an ALA Survey.* Chicago: American Library Association, 1981.

This report is the result of an ALA survey of publicly supported libraries which provide online search services using any of three vendors—BRS, DIALOG or SDC. Designed to answer questions such as, "should we charge users for online service?" and if so, "what costs do we consider when calculating a fee?" the report provides valuable data on costs which are included when calculating fees, fee structures, and percentage of direct costs paid by users. Appended is a "Supplemental Report on Fee Structures" and a discussion on the related literature, including fee-based services and no fee services. This source is extremely valuable in evaluating how other libraries are charging for online searches. The report is summarized by Lynch in *RQ* 21 (Spring 1982):223–6 and in *American Libraries* 13 (March 1982):174.

Matzek, Dick, and Smith, Scott. "Online Searching in the Small College Library—The Economics and the Results." *Online* 6 (March 1982):21–9.

The initiation of online search services in a small college library is described. A fee structure, differentiating service to faculty, students, administration and outside users, was established as an "artificial pricing plan," designed to "stimulate online searching." Benefits of online searching to the library include efficient answers to quick reference questions and generation of management data.

Penner, Rudolf J. "The Practice of Charging Users for Information Services: A State of the Art Report." *Journal of the American Society for Information Science* 21 (January-February 1970):67–73.

In a review of the literature, Penner indicates that libraries do not use sound costing principles (cost centers, billing systems, and cost-accounting systems) to determine costs for services, although larger libraries are moving toward that end. As of 1970, "society has not yet come to the point that paying for library information services is a common thing." This is a good review for historical purposes.

Popovich, Charles J., editor. *Fee-Based Information Services in Academic and Public Libraries. Drexel Library Quarterly* 19 (Fall 1983):1–92.

This thematic issue of the *Drexel Library Quarterly* is devoted to fee-based services. Articles by Ungarelli and Grant, Hornbeck, Reid, and Donnellan and Rassmussen discuss academic libraries, while articles by Gaines and Huttner, Tertell, and Woy discuss public libraries. Articles range from administration to examples based on successful operation of a fee-based service to surveys of information services.

Rettig, James. "Rights, Resolutions, Fees, & Reality." *Library Journal* 106 (February 1, 1981):301–4.

Fee-for-service, in particular for online searching, is discussed philosophically and morally (i.e., fees "violate the users' right of access to information"). Resolutions regarding fees are discussed. Realistically, fees are here to stay, and libraries should establish nondiscriminatory fee structures, such as making rates apply to all individuals as opposed to imposing fees or restrictions on groups or classes of users.

Rice, James G. "To Fee or Not to Fee." *Wilson Library Bulletin* 53 (May 1978):658–9.

A philosophical discussion of fees from the public library viewpoint, this article takes a practical stance on the subject. While free access to information is desirable, in reality it is better to charge for special services designed for specific patrons rather than restrict access by not offering these services at all.

Shannon, Zella J. "Public Library Service to the Corporate Community." *Special Libraries* 65 (January 1974):12–6.

The Minneapolis Public Library, in cooperation with the University of Minnesota Library and two other libraries, developed INFORM, a fee-based service for area businesses and industry. The progress, potential and problems of this project are discussed.

Waldhart, Thomas J., and Bellardo, Trudi. "User Fees in Publicly Funded Libraries." *Advances in Librarianship* 9 (1979):31–61.

This article reviews the economic aspects of library funding, the history of user fees, changing nature of library funding, input of new technologies and competition, and the philosophical debate on user fees. The authors conclude that public libraries, to fulfill their social objectives, must inevitably seek alternative sources of funding and that the impact of fees or equivalent systems needs to be explored.

Watson, Peter G., ed. *Charging for Computer-Based Reference Services.* Chicago: American Library Association, Reference and Adult Services Division, 1978.

A proceedings of a program organized by MARS, RASD, this group of articles presents "a broad, general review of some of the conceptual bases of a decision to charge or not charge," rather than a technical discussion of billing and accounting. The subjects of the three articles are: a history of charging for services in American libraries (Haynes McMullen), intellectual freedom and charging for computer based services (Zoia Horn), and the choices and implications of fees for online searching (Jan Egeland).

Watson, Peter. "The Dilemma of Fees for Service: Issues and Action for Libraries." *ALA Yearbook* 3 (1978):xv–xxii.

This is a practical discussion on the policies of libraries charging for online services. While the trend is toward charging for these services, the author discusses rationale to help librarians resist fees for online services.

Weaver, Carolyn G. "Free Online Reference and Fee-Based Online Search Services: Allies Not Antagonists." *Reference Librarian* No. 5/6 (Fall/Winter 1983):111–8.

The dual service philosophy, as espoused by the McGoogan Library, University of Nebraska allows for fees to be charged to users requesting online searches and simultaneously for free reference use of online databases. Online searches, which "are provided for the convenience and exclusive benefit of an individual," are considered a product, whereas use of online databases for reference is simply an alternative means of accessing information and therefore is a service.

Werner, Gloria. "Use of On-Line Bibliographic Retrieval Services in Health Sciences Libraries in the United States and Canada." *Bulletin of the Medical Library Association* 67 (January 1979):1–14.

A major part of this comprehensive study of online services

in health sciences libraries involves fee-for-service policies. In the study, 52.5 percent of the respondents charged for some or all of their services, while 47.5 percent absorbed all costs. The fee-for-service policies and average MEDLINE charges are broken down by type of institution and type of user.

INFORMATION BROKERS

Boss, Richard W. "The Library as an Information Broker." *College and Research Libraries* 40 (March 1979):136–40.

The author traces the history of the new information era, the emergence of information brokers, and the development of new technologies. Libraries can benefit from these new trends and work toward a national information policy. This paper previously appeared in *New Horizons for Academic Libraries* (papers presented at the first National Conference of the Association of College and Research Libraries), edited by Robert D. Stueart and Richard F. Johnson, New York, Saur, 1978, pp. 43–9.

Dodd, James B. "Information Brokers." *Special Libraries* 67 (May/June 1976):243–50.

Dodd presents an overview of the services provided by information brokers. These services primarily include photocopies and literature searches (both manual and computerized), but extend into non-traditional library services such as editing, speech writing, and indexing. Ethical issues discussed are conflict of interest, fees charged, and misrepresentation of work. Brokering is discussed from the view of the brokers themselves, libraries, and the end user. Information brokers fill a need for information services which, for a variety of reasons, libraries have not fulfilled.

"Information Brokers: Who, What, Why, How." *Bulletin of the American Society for Information Science* 2 (February 1976):11–20.

For this article, information broker is defined as an "individual or organization who—on demand—seeks to answer questions. . .and who is in business for a profit." Questions were sent to seven information brokers, asking what they do, who they serve, how the customer pays, what resources are used, etc.

Kalba, Kas. "Libraries in the Information Marketplace." In: *Libraries in Post-Industrial Society,* edited by Leigh Estabook. Phoenix, Ariz.: Oryx Press, 1977, pp. 306–20.

Libraries have not paid enough attention to the information marketplace, a major growth industry in the United States. New developments of special interest which place libraries under competition are special-interest magazines, online retrieval systems, and information brokers.

Maranjian, Lorig, and Boss, Richard W. *Fee-Based Information Services: A Study of a Growing Industry.* New York: Bowker, 1980.

Non-library-based, commercial information services represent a growing industry. These services are reviewed, with several major fee-based information services profiled. FIND/SVP is presented in detail. The chapter on marketing gives examples and suggestions for advertising.

Warner, Alice Sizer. "Information Services—New Use for an Old Product." *Wilson Library Bulletin* 49 (February 1975):440–5.

The formation of Warner-Eddison Associates, an independent information service in Massachusetts, is discussed very practically. Information brokers and possible competition with libraries is discussed along with the fee structure.

Warnken, Kelly. *The Information Brokers; How to Start and Operate Your Own Fee-Based Service.* New York: Bowker, 1981. (Information Management Series, #2.)

Warnken, Owner/Director of Information Alternative, has written a practical guide on how to start and operate an information brokerage, "from conducting an initial market study in the community, to setting up an office to the all-important key to success, getting and keeping clients." Included are an annotated list of potential services offered by brokers, practical advice on the "business" of running a business, and tips on building a clientele.

Index